Your

AGING

PARETNS

Sharm
Best regards.

Arriving at **Shared Solutions**
for Housing, Health
and Relationships

Maureen Osis and Judy Worrell

Maureen

Note for Librarians: A cataloguing record for this book is available from Library and Archives Canada at www.collectionscanada.ca/amicus/index-e.html
ISBN 1-4251-0796-6

Printed in Victoria, BC, Canada. Printed on paper with minimum 30% recycled fibre.
Trafford's print shop runs on "green energy" from solar, wind and other environmentally-friendly power sources.

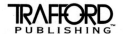

TRAFFORD
PUBLISHING™
Offices in Canada, USA, Ireland and UK

Book sales for North America and international:
Trafford Publishing, 6E–2333 Government St.,
Victoria, BC V8T 4P4 CANADA
phone 250 383 6864 (toll-free 1 888 232 4444)
fax 250 383 6804; email to orders@trafford.com
Book sales in Europe:
Trafford Publishing (UK) Limited, 9 Park End Street, 2nd Floor
Oxford, UK OX1 1HH UNITED KINGDOM
phone +44 (0)1865 722 113 (local rate 0845 230 9601)
facsimile +44 (0)1865 722 868; info.uk@trafford.com
Order online at:
trafford.com/06-2554

10 9 8 7 6 5 4 3 2

Contents

Benefits of this Book

Are you in the "sandwich generation"? Are you trying to find balance in your life, between the many competing demands of your own children, your work life, and your aging parents? If you are like most people your age, your life is very busy. You want direction – and you need it now!

Every family is unique. There are no "one-size fits all" solutions. This book is not a prescription. It is a guide to help you balance your life.

This book is written with you in mind. It will help you to think about the concerns and anxieties that you have about the older people in your life, and then suggest the steps to take to plan ahead and to find local resources that will work best for you and your family.

The book addresses the common dilemmas of

√   Health concerns: the physical, social, and emotional health of aging parents
√   Financial and legal concerns
√   Relationships: life-long relationships in the family and new demands as parents become frail or develop significant health problems
√   Living arrangements: the majority of seniors will continue to live in their own homes, and will need increasing support. Others will need to look at alternative housing options.

Information is empowering. With facts about aging families and suggestions for action, both generations can arrive at shared solutions for housing, health, and relationships.

How to Use this Book

This book is written in four sections, each containing three chapters. The book progresses from discussions about healthy aging and family relationships, to planning ahead, and considering shared decisions about financial and healthcare issues. It is not necessary to read the book in sequence – each chapter can stand alone. If there is a particular topic of interest, you can choose the parts of the book that will give you and your family some possible solutions. Each chapter includes useful links to resources, sources of additional information, and practical tips, checklists and action steps that can be taken by older adults and their families to address key concerns.

We begin with **Part 1 Understand Aging** to present the myths and realities of aging.

Chapter One How Ageism Hurts Us All describes how ageism and stereotypes about aging can be harmful. Interesting facts about Canadian seniors are presented. The chapter closes with practical tips for preventing the harmful effects of ageism.

Chapter Two Healthy Aging: Fact or Fiction describes the factors that affect normal aging, and how life satisfaction can be promoted in later life. The chapter concludes with tips for a healthy lifestyle during the aging process.

Chapter Three Everyday Realities of Aging: How Seniors Adapt provides a useful overview of changes related to aging processes, and how simple adaptations can allow continued activity and independence. The chapter includes helpful suggestions for supporting a parent with age-related changes in vision, hearing, balance, skin and sensation. In addition, the important topics of driving and medication management are discussed.

Part 2 Build Relationships talks about the importance of supportive relationships across generations, within the family and with health professionals when your parents begin to need services or healthcare.

Chapter Four Bridging the Gap: Understanding the Generations discusses how different generations' views of the world are shaped by events in their formative years, and how you can bridge the generation gap in your family.

Chapter Five Family Dynamics and Self Care raises crucial issues about the role of family members in providing help to parents – ideas to help you to know that you are doing the "right thing" and "doing things right" even from a distance. Suggestions for handling challenging situations and self-care are also included.

Chapter Six The Healthcare Team introduces the reader to commonly-used "medical jargon," and the members of the healthcare team across different settings. Ideas about communicating with healthcare professionals, and advocating for your parent are also provided.

Part 3 Plan Ahead addresses concerns related to health, finances, and housing. It explores how families can arrive at shared decisions about these important issues.

Chapter Seven Navigating the Maze: Finding the Services builds on the introduction to the healthcare team in the previous chapter. It gives a comprehensive overview of the types of public and private services available to seniors, and discusses how to go about finding these services. This chapter includes useful tips for arranging for services, in full consultation with your parent(s).

Chapter Eight Taking Care of Business: Financial and Legal Matters raises the sensitive topic of money and the personal costs of aging. Information about legal matters such as competency, guardianship, power of attorney, and healthcare directives is provided. Action steps and useful resources are included.

Chapter Nine The Meaning of Home discusses the deeply personal issues surrounding housing, and the importance of "moving by choice" rather than "moving by necessity." It has practical information about factors that make a "livable" community, and tips to help parents to stay at home. If this is not feasible, the chapter also has suggestions for making the decision to move, and helping parents choose the best option.

Part 4 Manage Health Concerns addresses many of the common chronic physical, and mental illnesses, as well as acute health concerns of older adults. It provides the reader with various strategies to support parents who are experiencing health problems.

Chapter Ten Chronic Illness: A Reality for Seniors discusses some of the common physical health problems, such as high blood pressure, heart disease, and arthritis. Ways to support your parent with these progressive, long-term conditions are included. Useful links to credible sources of information are also provided.

Chapter Eleven Challenges of Mental Illness presents an overview of common mental health problems. Practical checklists help you to identify symptoms, and take action when needed. Alzheimer disease and other dementias are also briefly addressed.

Chapter Twelve Acute Health Concerns provides a quick reference to acute conditions, which occur suddenly. It is designed to assist you to know when it is important to seek immediate or early treatment. Some of the conditions addressed include heart attack, stroke, and influenza. Risks of hospitalization and how you can prevent these are also included.

PART I

UNDERSTAND

AGING

CHAPTER ONE

HOW AGEISM
HURTS US ALL

Ask a teenager "Who is old?" and he or she will probably reply "Any-one over 30." Then ask the thirty something and you will likely hear "Seniors over 60." If you ask the senior, you will likely get another answer, such as "Any-one 10 years older than I am."

When teens forget, we think of them as uninterested or distracted. The forgetful adult is often called "stressed." - But seniors' lapses are labelled senility or "losing it."

Questions answered in this chapter:

What is ageism?
What are common myths of aging?
Who are Canada's seniors?
What is "aging anxiety"?
What can your family do to prevent the harmful effects of ageism?

This chapter dispels some common myths of aging, and reveals how ageism can hurt all ages. You and your parents can take action to avoid stereotyping the older generation.

What is Ageism?

Ageism refers to stereotyping and discriminating against or in favor of a particular age group. Robert Butler, who coined the term in 1969, explained that ageism highlights a few exaggerated characteristics of a particular age group and assumes that these qualities apply to everyone in that group.

How does ageism develop? With increasing mobility and other societal changes, very few families live in an intergenerational household. Some of you grew up with grandparents, but many others have had little exposure to the older generation and do not know what to expect as their own aging parents reach later life. In addition, increasing longevity has resulted in many more "old-old" seniors than ever before.

Erdman Palmore has written extensively about ageism, and he believes it is manifested in many ways. The following excerpt from his book entitled "Ageism" illustrates some examples of negative stereotyping:

Older persons falter for a moment because they are unsure of themselves and are charged with being "infirm."

Older persons forget someone's name and are charged with senility, and patronized.

Older persons are expected to "accept" the "facts of aging."

Older persons miss a word or fail to hear a sentence, and they are charged with "getting old," not with a hearing difficulty.

Older persons are called "cranky" when they are expressing a legitimate distaste with life as so many young do.

Edith Stein in *Ageism,* by E. Palmore

What are Common Myths of Aging?

What myths do you have about aging? Think about older adults you know who live in the community, not those who are in nursing homes or care centres. Decide whether you think the following statements are true or false.

Then explore the answers in this chapter.

T F About 80% of the aged are healthy enough to carry out normal daily activities.

T F The majority of older people have dementia.

T F The average older person cannot learn something new.

T F The majority of older people often feel miserable.

T F The majority of older people cannot adapt to change.

T F Many older people are isolated and lonely.

T F Life expectancy is longer for women then men.

T F The majority of older people live with family / spouse.

Health

If you were to ask your friends for their general perception of elderly people, many might describe the physical and medical disabilities associated with those who need care in a nursing home. This image overlooks the fact that about 80% of seniors aged 65 to 85 are healthy enough to carry on their daily lives and to participate actively in society. It should be noted, however, that many of those over 80 years do receive help, from family or friends, with at least one activity such as grocery shopping, housework, or money management.

Dementia

Many believe that it is inevitable for old people to have dementia, or cognitive impairment. This is not true. What are the statistics? Alzheimer Disease or other dementias affect 1 in 13 Canadians over age 65, although such afflictions are more common with advancing age.

Certainly, it is common to experience changes in memory with aging, as you well know when you search for your glasses or your keys! There is a modest decline in short-term memory, but this type of forgetfulness is normal and can be handled fairly easily by developing habits to keep track of things.

Dementia is much more serious than forgetting; it is a disorder that causes the individual to lose the ability to make decisions, to solve problems, and to conduct the activities of everyday life. (Chapter Eleven discusses dementia in more detail.)

Learning

You have probably heard that you "can't teach an old dog new tricks." The evidence shows that older people can continue to learn throughout their lifespan. Many begin new careers after "retirement." Many older citizens take on new challenges such as participating on their Condo Board, taking art classes, or volunteering at schools. Such activities can promote both social and physical health.

Life Satisfaction

Another common myth that you might believe is that older people are miserable, especially if you know someone who is. It is more likely that people who are miserable stay that way when they get old! The "old crank" was probably a "young crank" twenty years ago. Most seniors report that they are generally happy and satisfied with their lives, and some report that they are even happier now that the stresses of work and raising children are gone.

Adaptability

What about the common belief that old folks are stubborn and set in their ways? Think of seniors who have retired, moved from a house into a condo, traveled to foreign countries, adapted to physical changes and the loss of friends, and also kept current on the latest news. This describes many older people. Indeed, 13% of seniors' households in Canada have a computer in the home!

Isolation

Are older people isolated and lonely? This question is not so easily answered. Many older people are not lonely; they are still engaged in life and enjoying the companionship of friends. Social isolation, however, does tend to increase with age. Those who are widowed or experiencing serious health challenges are more likely to be isolated and lonely. They may be at risk for depression. (Chapter Eleven explores the effects of loneliness on mental health.)

Can you reconcile "ageism" with the following images?

John Glenn returned to space at the age of 77.

Michelangelo was carving the Rondanini just before he died at the age of 89.

George Bernard Shaw was 94 when one of his plays was first produced.

Well into her nineties, Canadian Doris McCarthy was still painting and traveling, and published her memoir, *Doris McCarthy: Ninety Years Wise.*

As Bette Davis said, "Old age ain't for sissies!"

Who are Canada's Seniors?

The term "senior" broadly refers to individuals over 65. There is a challenge when talking about seniors as a group; the term refers to people aged 65 to 95 and older. Other age groups cover a much smaller span. For example, the word "teen" refers to an age span of about 6 years! It is more helpful to think about older adults in three sub-groups: the "young-old" who are 65-74, the "mid-old" who are 75-84 and the "old-old" who are over 85 years of age.

The following overview provides a snapshot of seniors in Canada. We must remember, however, that there is a high degree of diversity among older adults.

Age and Life Expectancy

The population of Canada has been aging for several decades, and the increase in the proportion of those over the age of 65 will continue to grow considerably as a result of aging of baby boomers. At present about 12% of Canada's population is over 65 years of age.

The fastest growing age segment is the population 80 years and over. In Canada, for example, this group's numbers have increased by 41% between 1991 and 2001.

In 1997, the average life expectancy at birth was 75.8 for males and 81.4 for females; and at age 65, the number of expected remaining years was 16.3 for men and 20.1 for women. In the last 20 years, the difference in life expectancy between males and females has narrowed.

Gender

Elderly women outnumber elderly men, a margin that increases with advancing age. Women make up about 58% of those over 65 years of age and nearly 70% of those 85+.

Major Causes of Death

Among elderly Canadians most deaths are the result of chronic, degenerative diseases including heart disease, stroke, cancers, and respiratory diseases.

Marital Status and Living Arrangements

Senior men are more likely than senior women to live with a spouse. Approximately 77% of men over 65 live with a spouse, whereas only 44% of women do so. Among those over 65 years of age, 7% of men and 32% of women are widowed, and this increases among those 85+ to 39% of men and 79% of women. Senior women are much more likely to live alone and, as a result, are at greater risk for institutionalization.

Education

The current population of seniors did not have the educational opportunities that are present in today's society.

The level of education among seniors today is

- University degree: 8%

- Diploma or certificate: 12%

- High school - not graduated: 25%

- Grade 9 or less: 37%

Ethnocultural Variation

About 25% of seniors are immigrants, and most of them have lived in Canada for a long time (61% immigrated before 1961). At that time, the majority immigrated from Europe and other Western countries. In contrast, the majority of new Canadians today are from Asia, Africa, or the Caribbean. Seniors of the future will thus be much more ethically diverse. Immigrant seniors are more likely to live with extended family than Canadian-born seniors.

Paid and Unpaid Work

About 6% of seniors are in the paid workforce, and the majority of these are men. Those with university education are less likely to continue working. Employed seniors are more likely than other age groups to be self-employed.

The most common occupations among seniors are farming, sales, and management. About 25% of all seniors volunteer formally, and they spend an average of 3.9 hours per week doing so. In addition, 58% of seniors volunteer informally, usually in providing help and support to family and friends. A Canadian study found that three million retirees spent about five billion hours in volunteer service with an estimated economic value of $60 billion each year.

Seniors also make the largest charitable donations per annum of any age group: 80% make donations, often to places of worship.

Economics

The majority of seniors (68%) own their own home. Average income is $20,450, but women have a lower annual income than men ($16,070 for women compared to $26,150 for men). The main sources of income are OAS (Old Age Security), CPP/QPP (Canada/Quebec Pension Plans) and retirement pensions. Seniors spend about 59% of their annual income on food, shelter, clothing and transportation; 10% on recreation; 9% on household maintenance and furnishings; and 6-7% on health and personal care.

Activities

As many as 37% of seniors take part in weekly religious activities, 50% report being physically active on a regular basis, and another 12% report occasional physical activity. On average they spend 5 hours per day watching television.

What is "Aging Anxiety"?

Ageism is one of the many factors that contribute to our worries about growing older. Do you worry about growing older? If you answered yes, you are like many mid-life adults, or boomers, who experience aging anxiety for many reasons, including the following:

- living in a youth oriented society,

- observing aging parents with serious chronic illnesses,

- lacking knowledge about positive aspects of aging and adaptation, and

- experiencing age related changes as they approach 60.

Near the time of retirement we may begin to worry about future health and functioning as well as economic independence. Some of us fear changes in physical appearance associated with aging.

Aging anxiety affects both your attitudes and behaviour towards older people but it also influences your adjustment to your own aging experience. Knowledge about aging, such as the information that you will learn in this book, can help to alleviate your anxiety about growing older.

"When boomers are unnerved by the faces that stare back at them from the mirror, when their knees start to creak, when their sex drives do not drive them, or when they feel too stressed, or tired for sex, depression is not far behind. The generation who see themselves as changing the world must now face middle age, learning to live with losses and limitations while moving on with hope to new options."   Gloria Hochman

What can your Family do to Prevent the Harmful Effects of Ageism?

An ageist view of older people focuses on negative images. It assumes that they have less to live for, experience less joy, and are incapable of or have no desire to learn new skills. As with all stereotypes, these assumptions fail to recognize individual characteristics, positive tendencies and variation within the group.   You can stand up to this negative view by noticing the adaptability of older people. You will learn more about specific adaptations in Chapter Three: Everyday Realities.

Your aging parents may experience more overt ageism in their daily lives that causes them to feel out of the mainstream of society.   Having a sense of meaning and purpose in life is essential to emotional and mental health, and ageism erodes this sense of purpose.   Knowing more about factors that affect life satisfaction can help you to promote your parent's emotional and social well-being. You will find out more about healthy aging in Chapter Two.

Many seniors are more inclined than boomers to be cautious, traditional, and defer to authority so you may need to empower your parents to stand up for themselves.   You will read more about this in Chapter Four: Bridging the Gap.

Finally, ageism may cause you or your parents to avoid treatment for treatable problems on the false assumption that the cause of symptoms is "just a sign of aging" and nothing can be done. In Chapter Ten you will be reassured that many chronic health problems are treatable.

Useful Resources

For more information on Canada's seniors, visit the websites of

Statistics Canada at http://www.statscan.ca

Public Health Agency of Canada Aging and Seniors

http://www.phac-aspc.gc.ca

Take Action

This chapter has introduced the idea that ageism hurts everyone. Negative stereotyping dismisses the adaptability and accomplishments of the senior generation, and contributes to aging anxiety for the mid-life adult. Here are some actions that your family can take:

> ➤ Avoid being trapped in the myths of ageism – avoid stereotyping either generation!

> ➤ Learn more about aging by reading this book.

> ➤ Recognize if you have "aging anxiety" that might prevent you from seeing the positive aspects of aging.

> ➤ Talk about aging in your family, and focus on the positive aspects of getting older.

> ➤ Visit the website of ElderWise Inc. to read current information about health, housing, and relationships. http://www.elderwise.ca

CHAPTER TWO

HEALTHY AGING: FACT OR FICTION

Until recently most people believed that there was a pattern of aging that could be described as "normal." Most assumed that aging meant a decline in function and health. Now, we know that such decline is more related to lifestyle and physical activity than to aging itself. For example, osteoporosis is not a normal outcome of aging; it is loss of bone caused by a variety of factors some of which are under the individual's control.

What can we do to enjoy both a long and healthy life?

Questions answered in this chapter:

What factors affect aging?
What factors promote life satisfaction?
What are the top ten tips for healthy aging?
What can you do to help your parents enjoy healthy aging?

What Factors Affect Aging?

As you might assume, genetics play a role in aging and health, but according to the National Advisory Council on Aging (NACA), only about 30% of aging is determined by biology. Most of the changes that occur with age are associated with the following:

- diet and exercise habits,

- alcohol and tobacco consumption,

- psychological traits,

- and the presence or absence of support from family and friends.

Everyone wants to live long and to be healthy. No one wants to grow old, but what are individuals willing to do to offset the effects of aging?

The main threat to healthy aging is sedentary living. In Canada, for individuals over 80, death is usually preceded by 8-10 years of disability and about one year of dependency, which is often caused by a sedentary lifestyle. Although almost everyone agrees that regular physical activity is essential to good health, only about 30 – 40% of seniors actually engage in regular physical activity.

Heart disease is the most common threat to health for mid-life and older adults. Most disease and death due to heart disease could be prevented by physical activity and exercise.

What beliefs might impede involvement in recreational activities such as sports or fitness programs? Seniors might not place much value on leisure because a strong work ethic helped them to survive the depression, raise their children in post-war years, and save for a rainy day. Fear of injury is another common constraint; even young seniors are encouraged to "take it easy." Would you think of giving snowboarding lessons to a 65-year old?

What Factors Promote Life Satisfaction?

Life satisfaction can be thought of as the individual's personal assessment of progress toward his or her desired goals in life. As you would predict, poor health, loneliness, and financial problems decrease life satisfaction at any age. Did you know that seniors are likely to report the same levels of life satisfaction as younger adults?

Emotional Health in Later Life

Life satisfaction and emotional well-being are related. Geri Burdman, the author of *Healthful Aging*, described the five A's for emotional health.

- Appreciation: recognition from others and being needed

- Acceptance: the need to belong and associate with others with similar values

- Affection: paying attention to the happiness of others

- Achievement: having a sense of accomplishment

- Amusement: laughter, fun, and joy

As you read the components of emotional health, what came to mind regarding your own parents? Do they feel needed by others and by your family? Are they able to associate with others of their age and of similar interests? Do they get a chance to accomplish new things or to talk about the joys of their past accomplishments? And do they experience laughter – after all, "laughter is the best medicine."

Spiritual Journey in Later Life

The experience of spirituality is an individual journey that is related to, but differs from, religiosity. For some, spirituality provides a means of understanding death, a source of moral values, or a way of coping with suffering. For others, aspects of spirituality include hope, inner meaning, or a connection with transcendent love.

Spiritual activities may include praying, meditating, reading inspirational literature, listening to inspirational music, or participating in organized religion.

Older individuals look for meaning in aging. They want to understand why they are struggling with their loss of roles, identity, or capacity. For some, reminiscence and life review provide an opportunity to reflect on their life and legacy.

Social Well-Being

Social relations are fundamental to the experience of healthy aging. Roles give meaning and purpose to our lives. Researcher Carolyn Rosenthal found most families have important roles played by the older generation. One important role was that of the "Kinkeeper." Often a female, the kinkeeper is someone who works at keeping family members in touch with each other, thus maintaining stronger sibling relationships. The "Comforter" gives advice while the "Ambassador" represents the family at special occasions. Other roles were "Financial Advisor," Placement Officer (helps family members find jobs), and the "Head of the Family."

Supporting Life Satisfaction in Later Life

How can you support your parents' life satisfaction? What roles do your parents have now? How have their roles changed over the past five years?

Emotional and moral support are among the most common exchanges between parents and their adult children. You can encourage your parents to participate in family and social life through volunteerism, employment, social activism, family roles, and community involvement.

You may feel that this advice might not apply to your parents. You may be right. Before you suggest activities to your parents, you need to know their interests and personality.

What are the Top Ten Tips for Healthy Aging?

No known substance can extend life, but the chances of staying healthy and living a long time can be improved. Here are ten tips for healthy aging from the National Institute on Aging.

Top Ten Tips for Healthy Aging

1. Eat a balanced diet, including five servings of fruits and vegetables a day.

2. Exercise regularly.

3. Get regular health check-ups.

4. Don't smoke (it's never too late to quit).

5. Practice safety habits at home to prevent falls and fractures. Always wear your seatbelt in a car.

6. Stay in contact with family and friends. Stay active through work, play, and community.

7. Avoid overexposure to the sun and the cold.

8. If you drink, moderation is the key. When you drink, let someone else drive.

9. Keep personal and financial records in order to simplify budgeting and investing. Plan long-term housing and money needs.

10. Keep a positive attitude toward life. Do things that make you happy.

And if you want to add another, – floss your teeth daily! Yes, studies have shown that the practice of flossing teeth might extend your life and reduce the risk of stroke.

Useful Resources

Look for an opportunity to view the video series called "A New Look at Aging" (WHITE IRON Pictures, 2005).

The series is shown on Canadian Learning Television.
http://www.clt.ca

For more information on purchase, visit
http://www.distributionaccess.com

Read more about healthy aging. Visit Infoaging.org from the
American Federation for Aging Research (AFAR).
http://websites.afar.org

Take Action

Want to help your parents stay healthy?

> ➤ Next time you get together with your family, include
> a physical activity. Take a walk before supper. Play
> ball in the nearby park. Lift weights. Discourage your
> parents from engaging in "lazy living."

> ➤ Promote social well-being. Encourage your parents to
> maintain family roles and to take on new roles within
> their community.

> ➤ Take the list of "Top Ten Tips for Healthy Aging" and
> discuss with your parents. Which actions are they
> willing to do?

> ➤ Learn more about home safety to prevent falls.
> Chapter Three gives more information on this topic.

> ➤ Don't forget the mind! Engaging in new activities that
> are intellectually challenging actually stimulates new
> nerve connections in the brain. So start – or keep on –

> > • Reading
> > • Playing chess or bridge
> > • Joining a discussion group or book club
> > • Doing crossword puzzles
> > • Enrolling in a course

CHAPTER THREE

EVERYDAY REALITIES
OF AGING:
HOW SENIORS ADAPT

How can we help older adults to adapt to the everyday realities of aging?

As you read in Chapter One, there are many myths about how human beings age, both physically and mentally. This chapter considers the common age-related changes that affect everyday life. These changes are related to aging processes but occur at different rates for each individual.

There is no denying that these changes occur, but they do not have to cause great decline in activity and in quality of life. Sometimes very simple adaptations can allow your parents to continue an activity that they love indefinitely.

Questions answered in this chapter:

What are the everyday realities of aging?
Changes in
  vision?
  hearing?
  balance?
  skin and sensation?
When should we worry about our parents driving?
How can I help manage medications?
What are the risks of natural health products?

Everyday Realities of Aging

As noted in Chapter One, ageism can lead to negative ideas about aging. Chapter Two discussed factors that affect aging and life satisfaction. Some factors can be influenced by the individual's lifestyle. Other factors, such as genetics, are not under a person's control. What is under an individual's control is attitude and adaptation. This chapter reviews the many ways that seniors adapt and maintain quality of life despite age-related changes.

Changes in Vision

Several common changes occur in vision, Some are serious, while others require minor adjustments.

- The lens in the eye becomes yellow. This leads to difficulty in distinguishing blue from green. It is usually not a problem, unless the individual is an artist.

- The lens also loses some ability to change shape, which makes it harder to focus close up. This explains why so many people use reading glasses.

- The reaction time of the pupil slows down. This means it takes more time to adjust to light and darkness. Three times as much light is needed for reading or to do close work such as sewing.

- The perception of space may become distorted. This can affect driving.

- Some individuals lose some of their peripheral vision. This may lead to bumping into doorframes or other objects in the room. This loss can also affect driving.

Several eye diseases may increase with age: glaucoma, cataracts, and macular degeneration.

Glaucoma is a condition that causes greater pressure in the eye and can lead to blindness if not treated. Although is it not a normal part of aging, it is the most common cause of blindness among seniors. Medication administered in eye drops is the most common treatment although some individuals can be treated with laser surgery.

A *cataract,* or cloudy lens occurs in about half of seniors over 75 years of age. Often both eyes are affected. Cataracts are related to aging processes, but they occur at varying rates and degrees for different individuals. Treatment is surgical removal of the opaque lens and implantation of a clear plastic lens.

Macular degeneration is also related to aging. In this case, aging of the center (or macula) of the retina at the back of the eye occurs, and as the disease progresses, the centre of the field of vision is lost. Continued research is searching for prevention and treatment of this serious disorder.

Adaptations

Most individuals are willing to wear glasses to correct vision. Many are also willing and able to use eye drops to correct glaucoma and prevent blindness. Most seniors will accept cataract surgery and laser surgery when necessary.

Here are some other ways that people adapt to vision loss.

- They use a nightlight. Some lights are plugged into wall socket and shine a gentle light on the floor, showing a path from bed to the bathroom.

- They use a high watt or compact fluorescent bulb for reading or close work.

- They use magnifiers to read the phone book or to play cards.

Supporting a parent with vision changes

Here are some ideas to share with your parent.

To prevent or minimize vision loss:

- Have a yearly eye exam – this can lead to early detection of glaucoma, cataracts and macular degeneration.

- Wear dark tinted sunglasses in bright sunlight.

To treat glaucoma:

- Use eye drops faithfully.

- Watch for side effects of the medications and report to pharmacist or physician.

- Ask a pharmacist before using any over-the-counter medications. Some can worsen glaucoma by increasing pressure in the eye (antihistamines, for example).

- Buy a MedicAlert® bracelet to notify healthcare personnel of the glaucoma.

- Learn about activities that increase eye pressure and avoid doing these. (For example, lifting heavy objects).

To assist during cataract surgery:

- Cataract removal is done at day surgery. Your parent will appreciate your support before and after the procedure.

- Ensure that you have the correct eye drops and instructions prior to and after surgery.

Useful Resource

Visit the website of CNIB.

http://www.cnib.ca/vision-health

Changes in Hearing

Hearing is important to the quality of everyday living. It involves many aspects of day-to-day activities such as receiving directions, participating in conversations, listening to music, and enjoying recreation. Hearing loss can impact driving ability and safety.

For most seniors hearing loss is gradual. This slow change may mean that your parent is not aware of the change. Others in the family may notice it first. People with hearing loss often feel embarrassed by the inability to hear what is being said. This can lead to a sense of isolation and feeling depressed or frustrated.

The incidence of hearing loss in the older population is significant and increases with advancing age as follows:

- 65-74 years   25 – 30%

- over 85 years   50 - 60%

When you suspect hearing loss in your parent, suggest a hearing test. The best route is to begin with the family physician. The physician will check for infection or wax accumulation, which can significantly affect hearing. The physician can also refer to an audiologist for a hearing test. Your parent might be more willing to listen to this advice from the doctor than from you.

Supporting a parent with hearing loss

If your parent shows signs of hearing loss, here are some ideas.

- Ask your parent to talk to the doctor.

- Encourage a hearing test.

- Use the "Tips for Talking to Someone with a Hearing Loss" (see below).

- If your parent begins using a hearing aid, encourage patience. It takes time to get used to a hearing aid. Wearing it for a few hours a day at first may be helpful.

- Hearing aids increase the volume of voices but also of background noises, and that can take some adjustment.

- Look for ways to decrease background noise. When you are in the car, for example, turn off the radio.

- Consider using assistive devices such as telephone amplifying, TV and radio listening systems, and visual alerts such as a flashing light that indicates the doorbell. You can find out more about these devices from any audiologist.

> **Tips for Talking to Someone with a Hearing Loss**
> - Speak slowly and clearly.
> - Face the person while you are speaking.
> - Do not put your hands over your mouth. This muffles the sound. Also, some people use lip-reading when they lose their hearing.
> - Lower your voice, without speaking louder.
> - Reduce background noise and distraction.

Useful Resource

The Canadian Hearing Society http://www.chs.ca

Changes in Balance

Several changes in muscles and bones occur with age. These changes are more pronounced in individuals who are not active.

The large muscles in the legs reduce in size and in elasticity. This is one reason for morning stiffness. Another is that the joints become less flexible.

Bones lose their density and become more prone to fractures. The discs between each vertebra in the spine decrease in strength and width. This leads to a shortening of the spine, which explains why seniors lose some of their standing height.

With these changes in bone and muscle, there are changes in coordination. People may become less able to adjust their balance and are more likely to fall.

Note that arthritis is a very common disease. At least 55% of older adults report arthritis in one or more joints. For these individuals, tasks that require dexterous movements, such as buttoning a shirt, or picking up an object, can be difficult.

Adaptations

As people age, they slowly adapt their gait to adjust to changes in balance. They take shorter steps and place their feet wider apart. Many accept aids such as canes to ensure that they can continue to walk independently and safely. Others engage in regular exercise to maintain muscle strength and flexibility. Obviously, good shoes are important. And some attend classes with physiotherapists to learn specific exercises that improve balance.

Supporting a parent with changes in balance

The main focus in adapting to changes in balance is to reduce hazards in the environment that might increase the risk of falling. You could suggest some minor changes in the home. Offer to

- Locate an Occupational Therapist who will come into the home to assess risks in the environment.

- Contact a home healthcare agency, and ask for education on best ways to assist your parent to get in and out of a car, or up and down the stairs.

- Lower shelves and re-organize cupboards to avoid reaching.

- Release the tension on automatic door closers: heavy doors are hard to open and to keep open.

- Learn more about assistive devices, such as bathroom grab bars that contribute to safety. (See Useful Resource at the end of this section.)

See Chapter Twelve for more home safety ideas that help prevent falls.

Useful Resource

Visit the website of the Public Health Agency of Canada
http://www.phac-aspc.gc.ca

Follow the links by clicking on "Publications" and "Info-sheets for Seniors" and find "Assistive Devices Info Sheet for Seniors".

Changes in Skin and Sensation

While wrinkles are an obvious change in the skin, there are several others to note: the skin becomes more fragile and dry, wounds heal more slowly, and the colour and texture can change. Small harmless growths can appear anywhere on the skin, but there is also an increase in cancerous growths on the skin surface.

Older people are more prone to hypothermia – low body temperature. This is important in the Canadian climate.

Many people notice that the bones are more visible in an aging hand than in that of a young person. This change is due to the loss of fat (subcutaneous tissue) beneath the skin. This loss leads to the skin being more sensitive to heat and to cold. Fingers may lose some of their sensitivity to touch.

The foot experiences significant changes with aging due to changes in structure of the bones and muscles, and changes in circulation. Nails can become tough, brittle, and more difficult to cut. Generally, foot care is more challenging as older adults may have trouble reaching their feet. Because wounds will heal more slowly, good fitting shoes become very important at this age. Some structural changes can be treated by orthotics or surgery, for example:

• Hammer toes and bunions

• Fallen arches and metatarsal pain

• Plantar fasciitis

• Corns and calluses

Adaptations

Many seniors easily adapt to changes in the skin by using more creams or lotions to overcome dryness. They might bath or shower less often and use gentle soaps and shampoos. Using sunscreen is a good idea for everybody.

Some seniors are willing to wear "sensible" and good fitting shoes. Others will sacrifice comfort and safety for fashion.

Supporting a parent with changes in skin and sensation

You can help your parent to adapt to common changes.

- Remind them that new growths on the skin should be reported to their doctor.

- If you hear your mom or dad comment that your house is too cold you might need to adjust the temperature or keep a sweater or shawl handy when they visit.

- Have patience with those with arthritis in the hands. Simple activities take more time.

- Discuss the importance of avoiding heat exhaustion in summer. Increased sensitivity to heat may reduce the amount of time a senior should stay in full sun and heat. Watch the clock – don't stay out too long.

- Because wounds take longer to heal, encourage your parents to wear good shoes.

- Seek good foot care from a reliable professional. For example, some home care providers and nurse practitioners offer both basic foot care as well as specialized care for persons with diabetes.

Useful Resource

Visit the website of VON Canada, follow the links by clicking on "Health Education" and "Foot care"

www.von.ca

Worried about your Parents Driving?

The ability to drive gives people a sense of freedom and independence. For those seniors who have driven for their entire adult life, the loss of their license is a major threat.

Driving safety is affected by changes in vision and hearing, loss of muscle strength, flexibility, and slower reaction time. These changes don't mean that seniors have to turn in their driver's license at the age of 70. There are many adaptations that can prolong a safe driving record even into advanced years.

Adaptations

Many seniors acknowledge that their ability to make quick turns and read signs is reduced. Some will limit their driving to places they know well. Others will have someone else do the driving for a few trips, until they become familiar with the route and the potential hazards.

Because adjustment to light is impaired and night vision is reduced, many seniors restrict their driving to daytime trips. Further, some will watch road conditions, limit their driving to good weather roads, and avoid driving during winter storms or icy road conditions.

In some cases, though, senior drivers refuse to accept that their vision and reflexes have changed and believe that they are just as capable as ever. In this case, contacting the doctor may be necessary.

Supporting parents with driving

If you have concerns about your parent's driving, try these approaches to help both of you talk about driving, in a non-threatening manner.

- Remind your parent that you want everyone to be safe. Use the Questions About Driving Safety. (See page 30.)

- Take a drive with your parent. Watch for warning signs of unsafe driving. See the Checklist on Safe Driving. (See page 30.)

- Suggest changes such as limiting new routes, driving in the daytime, and avoiding tricky road conditions.

- Give gifts such as taxi vouchers to encourage your parent to use alternatives.

- Offer to pay for a driving education course. Avoid thinking that driving must end at a certain age. Remember, older adults can learn! Offer to take the course yourself. Many courses are now available for the Plus-55 driver.

- Encourage your parent to take driving lessons. Note that many older adults got a driver's license without ever taking any lessons. Be willing to take a refresher course yourself. Driving safely is in everyone's best interests.

Useful Resources

How to Care: Driving.
http://www.howtocare.com/driving.html

Additional resources can be found at www.elderwise.ca

 Visit the library page and look for the article titled "Your Aging Parents. Useful Resources."   This article includes all of the useful links found in this book.

If your parent agrees to talk about driving safety, use some of the following questions to begin the conversation. If your parent says yes to several questions, it might be time for a medical exam and/or driving test.

Questions About Driving Safety

Are you more nervous when driving?

Do you have frequent close calls?

Do other drivers honk at you?

Do you get lost when you are driving?

Do you find it hard to concentrate when driving?

Do any friends or relatives not want you to drive?

Did you get any traffic tickets or warnings lately?

Does your doctor think that you should be driving?

Take a drive with your parent. Watch for warning signs of unsafe driving. Use the following checklist. If you see several warning signs, talk to your parent about a medical exam and/or driving test. Note – if you are feeling brave, reverse the roles. You do the driving and ask your parent to check your safe driving habits.

Checklist on Safe Driving

Does the driver show any of the following warning signs?

☐ Drive too fast or too slow?

☐ Ignore or disobey street signs and traffic lights?

☐ Fail to yield to pedestrians or cars that have the right-of-way?

☐ Have trouble with highway ramps or merges?

☐ Make inappropriate turns (too wide or too sharp)?

☐ Have difficulty making safe left turns?

How can I help Manage Medications?

The majority of seniors take prescription or over-the-counter medications. Pain relievers are the most frequently taken, followed by drugs for high blood pressure, other heart medications, stomach remedies, diuretics (water pills), and cough or cold medication.

The use of medications is a double-edged sword! When used appropriately, drugs can relieve symptoms and benefit older adults; but with each medication used the risk of side effects and interactions increases.

Because elderly people may have several diseases, they may use many medications – a situation called *polypharmacy*. This puts them at risk for harmful reactions to drugs. Interactions between drugs or between food and drugs can cause further problems.

Older people do not metabolize and eliminate drugs as effectively as younger people. Some drugs stay in the body longer, and with repeated use can cause drowsiness or dizziness that can result in falls. In addition, if more than one physician is prescribing drugs, the risk of interactions may be overlooked.

Adverse drug reactions may be difficult to detect because symptoms such as confusion, dizziness, fatigue, or constipation are easily mistaken for medical conditions.

Terminology Related to Medications

Over-the-counter medication. Any medicine (drug) purchased without an order from a health professional.

Prescription medication. Any medicine (drug) that requires an order from a health professional, such as a medical doctor, pharmacist, dentist, or nurse practitioner.

Side effect. Any undesired effect that results from the action of the drug. Side effects are often predictable. For example, an aspirin may reduce headache but also cause upset stomach.

Adverse drug reaction. Any response to a drug that is unintended and harmful. These reactions may result in admission to hospital, danger to life, or prolonged treatment.

Adaptations
Many seniors appreciate that drugs can alleviate problem symptoms and improve their daily life. They are also aware that these same drugs can cause serious problems. They find ways to use medications safely.

- They use medications only when necessary.

- They do not take medications without a doctor's order.

- They consult with the pharmacist before taking an over-the-counter medication.

- When a new drug is added, they ask the pharmacist about interactions with other medications.

Supporting a parent with medications
You could encourage your parent to

- Use the same drugstore (or pharmacy.) The pharmacist will have accurate records of all the drugs that are being taken and can warn about possible interactions.

- Ask the pharmacist to package the medications in a blister pack or a dosette, a container in which the pills are placed in sections that clearly identify the dosage times.

- Contact the pharmacist if the pills do not look the same as those in the previous package.

- Follow the label instructions carefully. For example, can the drug be taken with food? Can it be crushed if your parent has trouble swallowing it? Some drugs are made to release slowly. Crushing the tablets will alter this property.

- Follow the recommended dosage schedule. Sometimes, when people forget a dose, they think that they should double the next dose. This could cause serious effects.

- Store medications in a cool, dry place, not the bathroom cupboard. Choose a cupboard in the kitchen, where the lighting is good to read the label, and grandchildren cannot reach the bottles.

- Watch the expiry date. Some drugs become toxic.

Here are some things you could do.

- Write out a schedule for your parent to check.

- Make a list of the medications for yourself. You will need this list if your parent is admitted to hospital.

- Make a note of all drug allergies. Encourage your parent to use a MedicAlert® bracelet, or to keep a wallet card noting the allergy.

- Check that your parent understands the medications. See the checklist – "What You Should Know About Your Medications" below.

Remember:

- All drugs cause side effects.

- Over-the-counter medications including vitamins, minerals, and herbal preparations or health-food supplements, may cause interactions and side effects. Encourage your parent to consult the pharmacist, physician, or other health professional before using these products.

What You Should Know About Your Medications

√ The name of the drug.

√ Why it is prescribed.

√ When and how it should be taken (with meals or not, whether alcohol or specific foods should be avoided).

√ What over-the counter-medications to avoid.

√ Side effects to watch for.

√ When to call the physician if adverse effects occur.

What are the Risks of Natural Health Products?

In Canada, the Natural Health Product Directorate regulates natural health products such as vitamins, herbal remedies, and homeopathic medicines. The goal of the NHPD is to "ensure that Canadians have ready access to natural health products that are safe, effective, and of high quality while respecting freedom of choice and philosophical and cultural diversity."

People sometimes confuse "natural" with "safe." Just because a product is natural does not mean that it is safe for anyone to take. Remember that both bacteria that cause illnesses, and fungi that can be lethal if eaten, are natural.

Willow bark, a product that is sold as a painkiller, is the original source for aspirin. Willow bark can also cause stomach pain, and when too much is taken, it can even cause stomach bleeding. Echinacea, a purple cornflower, is used in many remedies to help boost the immune system. If high doses are taken, however, it can cause nausea and dizziness.

Supporting a parent using natural health products

If your parent is using natural health products, there are things you can do/say to increase safety.

- Remind your parent that natural health products can interact with prescription medications. Check with the pharmacist.

- Note that natural health products that cause nausea or dizziness can have serious consequences for an older adult.

- Obtain natural health products from a reputable source. Check out credentials, and ask if the shop is registered with a provincial or national licensing body.

Useful Resource

Visit the website of the Public Health Agency of Canada http://www.phac-aspc.gc.ca. Click on "Seniors Health" and "Seniors Issues (Publications) to find several articles on "Medication Use."

National Health Products Directorate. http://www.hc-sc.gc.ca

Take Action

> Talk to your parents about their everyday realities of aging. Ask them about the adaptations that they are making in their day-to-day lives.

> Review the suggestions in this chapter and discuss with your parents. Perhaps you can add other adaptations that improve their quality of life.

> Usually, people will accept glasses easier than they will hearing aids. Often, they will say that they wish they had used a hearing aid sooner instead of becoming isolated from others. Find ways to suggest (gently) that your parent has a hearing test.

> Falls and resulting injury are a major risk for many seniors. Supporting your parent's adaptations to changes in vision, hearing, and balance can help to reduce the risk. Smart use of medications and herbal products can also promote safe living.

> Get to know your parent's pharmacist, a valuable member of the healthcare team. If you live at a distance, obtain the contact information, including e-mail or toll-free phone number so you can keep in touch.

> Regularly ask about medications!

Try this Quiz!

Here is one way to have a discussion on safe use of medications and herbal products. Make a copy of the quiz for your parents to complete. Compare everyone's answers.

Using Medications Safely

Indicate whether each statement is TRUE or FALSE.

1. Whenever possible, you should use herbal products instead of medications.

2. All drugs cause side effects.

3. Herbal products can cause side effects.

4. Polypharmacy means shopping at many pharmacies.

5. Store your medications in the bathroom cupboard.

6. If you forget to take a dose of medicine, you should double the dose next time.

7. Over-the-counter drugs are safe for everyone.

8. Always purchase your drugs from the same pharmacy.

9. It is okay to use drugs after their expiry date.

10. If you have trouble swallowing pills, crush them and mix with food.

Here are the answers to the quiz, with the chapter pages.

1. False, page 34

2. True, page 33

3. True, page 33

4. False, page 31

5. False, page 33

6. False, page 32

7. False, page 33

8. True, page 32

9. False, page 33

10. False, page 32

Note: you can download this quiz from the ElderWise website and e-mail to family or friends. Visit the Library page to find the quiz. www.elderwise.ca

PART 2

BUILD RELATIONSHIPS

CHAPTER FOUR

BRIDGING THE GAP:

UNDERSTANDING THE GENERATIONS

A generation refers to a group of people who are approximately the same age. Each generation or cohort is shaped by the significant events occurring in the world around them during their formative years. Because of these common influences, the group develops its own collective personality and attitudes about authority, work, and family.

Perhaps you have noticed the generation gap in your family; for example when you suggested that your mother hire someone to clean the house, she replied; "Money doesn't grow on trees!"

Questions answered in this chapter:

How do different generations view the world?
What are the generation gaps?
How can we bridge the generation gaps in our family?

How do Different Generations View the World?

Did you know that the term "generation gap" first arose in the 1960's to describe the many differences such as taste in music, fashion, and politics between the baby boomers and their parents? Now, over forty years later, there exists a new generation gap – the differences in experience, opinions, behaviour, and expectations between adult children in their 50's and older adults in their 80's. Understanding the key generational differences is helpful in promoting acceptance and avoiding conflict between generations within families.

As the population ages, the number of generations is expanding. In this chapter, we will explore the worldviews of three main groups that have been labeled builders, boomers, and busters.

Builders or Veterans: b. 1925 - 1945

The builders or veterans were born from approximately 1925 to 1945 and grew up in difficult times as they experienced world wars, the Great Depression, and the atomic bomb. How often do you hear veterans speak of the hardships encountered during the Depression? This was an event that left an indelible mark on many of today's seniors and may explain why they place such importance on savings. They are traditional in their views and value commitment, dedication, duty and sacrifice. They were taught that authority should be obeyed. Family life was important, and Mother was most likely a homemaker. They were most influenced by family and church. In contrast to the economic challenge of their youth, many joined the new middle class during their working years. These are the seniors in our population, the parents of baby boomers.

Baby Boomers: b. 1946 - 1964

The boomers, born between 1946 and 1964, are the largest cohort in history. Unlike their parents, they are more focused on self-fulfillment than on duty, and they tend to challenge authority. Boomers grew up in a time of prosperity and thus developed a sense of entitlement. They experienced the Cold War, the Civil Rights Movement, the Viet Nam War, and Feminism. Family life had to manage through divorce, remarriage, and two working parents. Boomers are most influenced by family and education. They equate work with personal fulfillment and expect respect from subordinates. There are 10 million Canadian baby boomers - one third of the population. As of 2007, the first wave of the boomers turns 60! To find out what kind of boomer you are, refer to the box on the next page.

Baby Busters: b. 1965-1983

The baby busters, or Generation Xers were born between 1965 and 1983. This group has experienced rapid change in social and family structures, notably the rise of working, single mothers. Unlike their workaholic parents, busters are more skeptical about work, particularly regarding job security. They tend to be self-reliant and value peer relationships and work-family life balance. They witnessed the fall of the Berlin Wall, the Persian Gulf War and the spread of AIDS. They demand balance between work and personal life. They are most influenced by the media and friends.

What Kind of Boomer are You?

If you are an <u>early boomer</u> you were born between 1947 and 1951. You are seriously thinking of retirement but probably cannot afford to, just yet. You may still have children at home, either teen-agers or "boomerang" kids who have returned. You long for the "empty nest" which rarely exists anymore. You will be among the first of the aging boomers, turning 75 sometime between the year 2022 and 2027. You were between 9 and 13 when the sixties began: you probably remember much of the social change during that time.

If you are a <u>middle boomer</u> you were born between 1952 and 1958. Retirement is a long way off, and you are still raising your family. You were between 2 and 8 years of age during the turmoil of the sixties. Too young to be part of the social movement, you might remember it through the media, or from the stories told by your older family members.

If you are a <u>late boomer</u> (not bloomer), you were born between 1959 and 1966. Do you even identify yourself as a boomer? When the first boomers turn 75 in the year 2022 – you will be between 57 years and 62 years of age – and probably still working.

Sandwich Generation

The term "sandwich generation" was coined to describe the experience of being caught in the middle of two generations. Many of today's boomers know the experience of worrying about their parents, who are in their 70's and 80's, and at the same time, involved with their children, who might be teen-agers and young adults. They assumed they would experience an "empty nest" as their children left home; instead, they have the "boomerang kids." These young adults return home because of pressures of finances or health.

What are the Generation Gaps?

Where do your family members fit in these generational layers? Of course, these are only general descriptions, for within each generation considerable variation may exist! Each generation, however, is influenced by culturally defined expectations. For example, veterans were expected to marry young and have children. Baby boomers tended to leave home in their late teens, and they often pursued education and/or career responsibilities before marrying and having children. The socially - defined timetables are shifting as younger generations remain in their parents' homes for longer periods of time and, if they marry and have children, do so at much later ages than in previous generations.

Consider how each generation has come to view the world as a result of world events at important developmental periods in life. For the traditional builders, the hardships experienced during childhood have contributed to the view that you should be grateful to have a job. They believe in saving for the future. There are black and white answers in their modern view of the world, which evolved during the scientific era.

Baby boomers, like their parents, grew up when science prevailed, and they too hold a modern view, but they are more inclined to spend rather than save (with a credit card, not cash) and are more individualistic than their sacrificing parents. The baby busters had to become self-reliant and deal with greater diversity, so they tend to view the world as gray rather than black and white.

In the following descriptions let's assume that your parents are veterans, you are a baby boomer, and your children are busters.

When you think about your parents do you see some of the characteristics of veterans?

- Do your parents view family life as highly significant?

- Do they expect commitment and dependability from you?

- Have you noticed hierarchical, almost militaristic views? Expectations based on gender stereotypes?

- How do they feel about using their hard earned savings to pay for services?

- Do they bow to authority figures, such as the physician or healthcare administrator?

- Do they follow the rules and regulations?

When you think of yourself, do you share the characteristics of baby boomers?

- Do you sometimes feel your parents expect too much of you because they believe that families should help and support one another?

- Are you worried that increasing responsibilities for family care will have a negative impact on your work or pension?

- Do you sometimes find it difficult to balance your work life with your family life?

- Does it bother you that there are so many rules, regulations, and eligibility criteria for services for seniors?

When you think of your adult children, do you see the characteristics of busters?

- Do your children seem too concerned with their own lives and friends rather than with family?

- Is their communication sometimes abrupt?

- Do they maintain contact with your parents on their own or do you need to initiate this?

- Do you think that your children are too self-centered and uninvolved in your life?

- Do you worry about their lack of drive when it comes to work and career?

- Do you find that your children don't want you to tell them what to do or take your advice?

How can we Bridge the Generation Gaps in our Family?

Comparing the general beliefs, values, and life views of the three generations can help you bridge the gaps in your family.

Consider the following communication principles when having family discussions.

- Listen actively to what others are saying – give them feedback about their opinions by asking them to validate your understanding of their meaning. Ensure also that others comprehend what you say.

- Suspend your own judgments when listening.

- Pay attention not only to "what" is said, but also to "how" it is said and what is "not stated."

- Watch body language (facial expressions, posture, tone, gestures) that might add to the meaning of the message or contradict what a family member actually says.

- Show that you are paying attention – maintain eye contact, nod, respond.

- Remove barriers to listening – distractions, preoccupation, and self-talk.

- Ask open ended questions – these are questions that cannot be answered with a simple "yes or no" – many begin with "how, why, or what."

For ideas on having family conversations, see the box below.

Family Conversations: Talking About Your Differences

What was a defining moment in history for you?

When you were a teenager, what were some of the fads? Clothing styles?

Who was your favourite movie star when you were growing up? Television program? Music group?

What can you teach us in our generation?

What do you think that you can learn from other generations?

Think about the following suggestions for connecting the generations.

Bridging the Generation Gaps

- Make a unexpected telephone call: focus on checking in – not checking up

- Send a long distance telephone gift card

- Write a letter -- with today's high-speed world and increasing use of e-mail, we forget the pleasure of finding personal mail in our box

- Take a road trip together: use the time to get to know each other in the present moment – and enjoy the surprise of finding out new things about each other.

Take Action

> ➤ Have an open conversation with your parents. Let them know that you understand their views and values. Some ideas are presented below.

Mom and Dad – I want to say...

You have experienced major changes in your lifetime, and so have I.

Some of your views are different from mine and that's okay.

You grew up in a more traditional time, and I value some of our family traditions.

You worked hard to achieve what you have gained, and so have I.

You have a wealth of experience and knowledge; me too.

You have the ability to make decisions and choices as do I; you respect authority, but I don't to the same degree.

I really care and want to do the right thing.

> ➢ Have a conversation with your children who are
>   probably young adults, and members of the baby
>   buster generation. Some ideas are presented below.

To my children, I want to say...

You are driven by different things than I am, and I am trying
to accept that.

You care about work-life balance, and I wish I could pay
more attention to this.

You are self-reliant and do not want to be controlled, and I
try not to give you advice.

You don't care for too much structure or unnecessary rules,
and I can see your point.

You are serious about life, and I am proud of your adult
accomplishments.

I really care and want to do the right thing.

CHAPTER FIVE

FAMILY DYNAMICS AND SELF CARE

Charlotte Eliopoulos, a noted Gerontological Nurse, writes "a family is a strong chain of human experience that bonds its members together through life's challenges and joys."

Whether united through challenges or joys, many family relationships are complex. The sense of duty and obligation toward parents may differ depending on the family's culture and beliefs and on individual expectations.

Societal expectations also impose certain norms and a sense of obligation toward family members. And, as the healthcare system evolves with cost containment and reduction of services, there is a growing expectation that families will provide what the healthcare system does not.

Questions answered in this chapter:

How can I know when my parents need help?
Do I have role reversal?
How do I figure out the right thing to do?
How do I provide support from a distance?
How do we handle challenging situations?
How do I take care of myself?

Most people have several roles or functions – son/daughter, sibling, spouse, parent, teacher, etc. These roles define who you are and also determine the responsibilities that you carry. For example, if your children are still living at home, you will have more responsibility attached to your parenting role than if they are living independently.

Modern life is busy, - and people experience competing demands. When you begin to consider if your parents need your help, you may initially feel a bit overwhelmed and wonder how you can manage it all. On the other hand, you may also feel a sense of obligation to your parents. After all, they cared for you early on in your life, and now it is time to reciprocate and offer your support.

How do you feel about this? How will this added responsibility affect your other roles and responsibilities? Do you have enough time, energy, and personal resources to take on the helping role?

Be proactive and talk to your parent(s) about their wishes, expectations, and from whom they want to receive help. It is far easier to have these important conversations before the fact, rather than when an urgent need arises.

How can I Know when my Parents Need Help?

In families with close relationships, the parents and adult children discuss changes that occur with aging and transition. They talk about the future and share expectations about supporting each other. Many older adults, however, do not want to be a burden to the younger generation and might not ask for support. Because changes in health might be slow and gradual, it is sometimes difficult to determine when help is needed.

What are some signals that might indicate to you that your parents need help?

- Safety concerns arise. A parent has unexplained bruises, trips or falls, and driving is a concern.

- Others, neighbors or relatives, express concern about your parents.

- Forgetfulness and confusion are more apparent; for example, a parent forgets to turn off the stove or to take medications, misses appointments, fails to pay bills, or becomes lost in familiar territory.

- Personal hygiene is not at the same level as before.

- You are worried that your parent isn't eating nutritiously (weight gain or loss).

- Your parent is isolated, not as sociable as in the past, doesn't go out much.

- Household maintenance and housekeeping are deteriorating.

- Your parent is showing changes in mental or emotional health; for example, he or she is more irritable or shows changes in personality.

- You notice an increased use of alcohol.

If you notice these warning signs, try to spend more time with your parents and notice day-to-day coping. If you live at a distance, talk to others who live closer. Do they share your worry?

Do I have Role Reversal? Do I become my Parents' Parent?

When the question of role reversal is posed to experts, the universal answer is an unequivocal "NO!" If your parents need help, some of the new responsibilities may seem like those of parenting; but your parents will always be your parents, and you will always be their child. They are adults with a wealth of experience, and well-established ways of coping with life's challenges. If you assume the role of "parent," this may impose a sense of control or authority over the parent and result in conflict in the relationship. Recognize this, and treat your parent with the respect you would offer any other adult, regardless of any physical or cognitive infirmity they may have.

How do I Figure out the "Right Thing" to do?

Many adults worry more as their parents age; they want to do the "right thing," but they are not sure what is "right." When you notice that your parents are showing signs of frailty or decreasing capability in managing the affairs of daily life, you might be tempted to rescue them. For example, you might urge them to move closer to you, with the good intention of being more available to them. Will such a decision work in everyone's best interests?

Spend some time thoroughly assessing exactly what is underlying the need for help. Has there been an acute medical event (heart attack or stroke), or are the long-term effects of chronic illness affecting your parent's ability to care for him or herself? Be specific about the type and amount of assistance that is needed to support your parent. Sometimes, minimal help with very specific tasks can make a profound difference! Remember, the key is to maintain independence and autonomy for your parents for as long as possible.

Here are some ideas to help you know that you are doing the "right thing" and "doing things right."

Respect and protect privacy. Some conversations may involve sensitive issues such as financial information and personal health history. Engage in respectful conversations with your parent, siblings, and other important people in your parent's social and support networks. These discussions may be difficult, as everyone will likely be experiencing various degrees of uncertainty, anxiety, and stress brought on by the changing circumstances and role relationships.

Accept differences. Remember the generation gaps! You and your parents may have different values, opinions, and attitudes. Be sensitive to differing views, and recognize that not everyone will feel the same.

Nurture self-esteem. Quality of life is subjective and means different things to different people, but one common element is the need for meaning in life - to feel useful and valued by others. Self-esteem is nurtured with praise, encouragement, and recognition of the ways in which someone adds to your life. Try to do this in every encounter.

Involve significant others. Include those people in your parents' networks who care about them. These people can provide strength and may be willing help out in ways that you might not have considered. Maintaining social contacts and interests improves the quality of daily life for older adults, as it does for anyone.

Foster independence. Offer choices and always allow full participation in decision making and planning. Even people with mild to moderate cognitive impairment can make some decisions and express their preferences.

Sometimes, you just need to do something! You might not have a choice and need to step up to the plate and help out. In the case of a medical emergency, it is relatively easy to know what needs to be done. In the case of a slow decline, however, things are not as clear-cut, and you need to be careful not to over-react and take over where there is no undue risk to others.

How Do I Provide Support from a Distance?

Family relationships and personal choice will in part determine how you provide support to your parents. Proximity will also determine how you do this. If you live some distance from your parents, your role will be more challenging (see tips on page 56). In addition, financial resources will dictate the extent to which paid services can be utilized, for example, hiring someone to do yard work or housekeeping.

Tips for providing support from a distance

Maintain contact

- Visit as often as you can; plan ahead to make the best use of your time.

- Phone frequently; set up a schedule.

- Encourage others to call; set up a rotation schedule for checking in.

- Set up easy lines of communication such as email or fax.

- Develop a secure family website to keep in touch.

- Offer to pay for these communication tools as special occasion gifts.

Learn as much as possible about your parent's community

- Who are their neighbours? Will they respond in time of need? Will they give you their phone number and take yours for emergencies?

- Find out what services are available, such as gardening, household maintenance, housekeeping and transportation.

- Use community resources (senior centres, meal delivery, transportation, adult day care).

- Organize local support (neighbor, friend, church).

- Hire people to assist with specific tasks.

Protect your peace of mind

- Make a list of important documents, including health care directive, personal health and insurance numbers. (See Chapter Eight for more information.)

- Keep important phone numbers and contacts in a binder.

- Consider a personal emergency response system. (See page 84.)

How do we Handle Challenging Situations?

How Do I Get Help From Others in my Family?

Usually, one person in a family assumes more responsibility for supporting aging parents. Often, this is the adult son/daughter who lives closest. Siblings who are geographically distanced may feel guilty for their inability to help.

Often, brothers and sisters may get along well but still not see eye-to-eye when it comes to concerns about their parents.

Consider having a family meeting, including your parents, to explore everyone's worries. Establish an air of open acceptance and honesty. Set an agenda for the meeting and don't forget to talk about things that are going well.

What do I do if Parents Will Not Accept my Help?

Initial discussions can be difficult, especially if your parents do not see the need for help, or they are unwilling to accept help because they don't want to be a burden. People need to feel that their relationships are two-way, so if you can find ways to show your parents how they are giving something to you in return for your assistance, they may feel a greater sense of reciprocity and be more inclined to accept your help.

They may be worried that getting help means a loss of independence. Try to discuss this topic when it is a "future possibility." Ask your parents how they want to handle future needs for support. You may need to obtain more information about alternatives and what services are available in your parent's community so that your parent is making an informed choice.

Some individuals refuse help because of mental or emotional disorders. If your parent has addictions to alcohol or drugs, he/she may not willingly accept your advice. If your parent has a long-standing mental health disorder, again advice for treatment may be rebuked. If you are caught in one of these distressful situations, you might find help in the resources mentioned later in this chapter or through professional counseling.

As noted earlier, it is important to involve others in these discussions. If someone else notes the need for help and confirms what you have been saying, your parents may be more inclined to agree. They may listen more closely to their peers or prefer to have friends help out rather than ask you to do so at this time.

At the end of the day, you must respect a parent's decision even if you do not agree with it. Unless there is a major risk to others, or your parent is not competent to make decisions because of a medical diagnosis, your parent has the right to choose.

How do I Set Limits?

Another challenging situation occurs when your parents have unrealistic expectations of you, and you are unable to provide the extent and type of assistance that they desire. In this case, it is important to be clear on your role, and in your conversations with your parents specify what you can and can't do, when and where you can provide help, and how much time you can spend. Once you have set the limits, stick to them. Don't be persuaded "just this once" because your indecision will be evident, and the unrealistic expectations will continue.

Be aware of the impact on your other relationships and roles, especially with your spouse and children. If you are still working, you may need to plan ahead and discuss this situation with your employer or the human resources department to see what kind of support and assistance might be available in your workplace. Check out your employment benefits to determine if they include the provision for elder care. Depending on your job, you may have other options for increased flexibility in your work role. You may need to let go of some of the things that can wait. Focus on the really important things in your life.

Don't try to do everything alone. Sometimes, this situation requires a family meeting to talk about options and ways in which others can share the load.   Chapter Seven provides more information on finding services and support.

How do we Handle Family Conflict?

Sudden changes in health, hospitalization, or a move into a long-term care centre for one of your parents can precipitate a family crisis. Crisis situations are turning points. Families either negotiate the challenges and move on or fail to negotiate with resulting distress.   The crisis is caused, not solely by the problem, but also by the inability of the family to cope effectively using their usual problem-solving methods.

Crisis

Taken from the Greek work "krinein," it means to decide. From the Chinese characters, crisis means "danger" because it threatens to overwhelm and "opportunity" because during times of crisis, individuals and families may experience growth and increased competence.

If your family has open communications and strong, healthy family ties, you will manage the changes and challenges. But what if your family has a long history of difficult relationships, and communications are challenged by mental health disorders or clashes in personalities?

What can you do if you are caught in family conflict, either between yourself and your parents or among your siblings?

First and foremost, acknowledge unresolved family issues. If you did not get along well with your parents and/or siblings in the past, it would be unreasonable to expect this to change because they need your help. Try to identify and address unresolved issues honestly and in a realistic manner. If possible, engage in respectful discussions about things that are troublesome. Become aware of your own reactions. You may need to lower your expectations about the extent to which change is feasible and accept your family members as they are. At times, families need professional counseling to help them work through their unresolved issues.

Avoid roadblocks or triggers. Triggers may be rooted in automatic responses in the family that have little to do with the present situation. Most families develop repetitive and predictable communication patterns – an automatic response that comes out in stressful situations. Some patterns can be helpful; others can be unproductive, especially when one member does not have his/her needs met.

Here are some responses that block communication:

• False reassurances – "Everything will be okay, Mom"

• Giving advice – "If I were you, I would ..."

• False inferences – "What you really mean is ..."

• Moralizing – "It is wrong to ..."

• Value judgments – "That wasn't the right way to ..."

• Superficial social responses (clichés) – "That's nice, Mom"

Practice reflective listening. Listen to what your family members say, and do your best to understand what they are feeling. Try the following steps:

• Ask a family member to clarify if you don't understand.

• Be empathic and reflect the feelings that underlie the words.

• Be concrete and stay relevant.

• Guard against making assumptions.

Reflective listening is demanding and you might not be able to do it if you are too emotionally involved or exhausted.

Manage issues. Within your family, establish a method for handling disputes, and if possible, deal with issues one at a time. Sometimes you need to start with issues that are easiest to resolve or break down a big issue into manageable chunks. Try to find a solution that meets everyone's basic and legitimate needs.

Follow the steps of collaborative problem solving. This approach is helpful in finding solutions that are acceptable to everyone. No one loses, and everyone benefits.

1. Define the problem in terms of needs.

2. Brainstorm possible solutions.

3. Select the best solution that will meet the needs of all.

4. Make a plan (who, what, where, when) and implement the plan.

5. Evaluate the outcome and make adjustments, as necessary.

How can I Take Care of Myself?

This chapter began by noting "family relationships are complex." For some families, the complexity arises out of conflict. For others, the new role of responding to the changing needs of aging parents creates confusion and uncertainty. Unfortunately, some individuals have had to cope with unhealthy family dynamics all of their lives.

If you are reading this book, you want to find shared solutions to common concerns in collaboration with your parents. The role that you play may fall along a continuum from occasional support to daily interaction. Depending on your level of involvement, you might be at risk for fatigue, emotional distress, or burnout.

Self Care

Expect emotional challenges – you are striving to do your best. You will experience challenges and difficult situations as you assume more responsibility in your new role. There is much to learn. Be kind to yourself and know that you are doing the best you can.

Enjoy life and try to find something pleasant each day. Sometimes life's simple pleasures are forgotten in the "busy-ness" of daily life. Try to find something pleasant each day and share these pleasures with your parents. Humour is a great tension reliever and can sometimes effectively turn a potentially negative situation into a positive one.

Use assertiveness. This communication style allows you to maintain self respect, and have your own needs met without dominating or ignoring the needs of others. Messages with three parts are helpful. The three parts are

- o   a behaviour (when you do …),
- o   a feeling (I feel …) and
- o   an effect (because it causes me …).

For example, perhaps you need to assert your need for more advance notice when your mother phones and asks you to take her to see a physician because she often calls at the last minute with this request. You could say something like this. "Mom, when you call me at the last minute to take you to the doctor, I feel really strapped for time. I have to call my boss at home in the evening, or catch him first thing in the morning to reschedule my work for the day in order to take the time off."

Self Care for Challenging Situations

If you are an adult child of an alcoholic parent, you will know that your family is not likely to address problems openly. The addiction may be a carefully guarded family secret. Families who are faced with this frustrating situation might be tempted to cut-off from the parent.

If your parent has a newly-diagnosed mental health disorder, such as depression, this may present challenges to the family. For example, depression tends to affect judgment, memory, and self-esteem - all required for healthy decision-making. See Chapter Eleven for more information on the challenges of mental health.

If your parent has a chronic and persistent mental health disorder such as schizophrenia or bipolar depression, you know that these disorders continue in later life. Effective treatment is essential to prevent relapses.

If your parent has personality characteristics that cause distress or damage interpersonal relationships, then your journey with your aging mother/father will be more difficult. You will likely be caught between wanting to be helpful to your parent and wanting to take care of your own mental health. Ageism may contribute to your sense of being trapped. Society, including many health professionals, may have the attitude that you owe respect to your parents, that you must not abandon them. This view overlooks the responsibility that the older person has for his/her own behaviour. And it also ignores your need to protect yourself from a potentially harmful relationship.

If you are experiencing emotional abuse from your parents you may need support to stop the abuse. The abuse might be a life-long pattern of interpersonal behaviour or a new pattern occurring because of the onset of mental health problems.

To avoid abuse, you need to recognize it. Emotional abuse occurs when one person controls another through the use of fear, criticism or manipulation.

Steps for Self-care in Challenging Situations

If you have *any of the above problems* in your life, you need to take care of yourself. *Don't try to do this alone.* Here are some steps you can take.

One: Talk to a social worker who is in a geriatric program. There may be an outreach program that can make contact and encourage your parent to seek treatment.

Two: Consult a lawyer regarding competency; look for a lawyer with Elder Law interests and credentials.

Three: Attend a program to learn more. For information about addictions, contact Al-Anon in your community. Al-

Anon is an organization for those whose lives have been affected by someone who abuses alcohol. Al-Anon teaches people to detach and to release themselves from responsibility for another person's disease or recovery.

Four: Learn to set healthy boundaries. Boundaries are the personal limits that we set with other people that tell others how we will let them treat us. Boundaries are not about controlling others but about what we need in order to take care of ourselves. Without boundaries, we lose the sense we have of ourselves.

Useful Resource

For information about acute or chronic mental health disorders, contact the Canadian Mental Health Association. http://www.cmha.ca

Take Action

- ➢ Notice the signs that your parents need more help or support, but don't jump in without asking their permission.

- ➢ Respect family roles. No matter what your parents need, they will always need you to be their son/daughter. Don't fall into the trap of thinking that you become their parents!

- ➢ It's always hard to know the right thing to do for others. Talking about concerns and sharing the decisions can help to get it right.

- ➢ Don't do it alone! Reach out for information, support, and encouragement from others, including family, friends, community, and professionals.

CHAPTER SIX

THE HEALTHCARE TEAM
WHO ARE THEY?
HOW CAN WE INTERACT?

The healthcare team varies with the setting. If your parent is hospitalized, you and your parents will interact with many different professionals, each with a unique and specialized role.

In the community, you and your family will most likely meet homecare – or community-care nurses. You might also meet other specialists such as social workers, physiotherapists, or occupational therapists.

Questions answered in this chapter:

How can we understand medical jargon?
Who are the members of the healthcare team?
How can we interact with the team?
How can we advocate for our parents?

Care of older adults is complicated by the interaction of aging processes and disease. Good healthcare is a very complex process involving many different health-care providers, and aging parents often need the support of health professionals. Getting to know the members of the health-care team can be a daunting task.

Usually an interdisciplinary team is involved, with each member playing a specific role. The term "interdisciplinary" refers to the composition of the team; many different disciplines come together to assess, diagnose, and treat the common health problems that occur for older adults.

How can we Understand Medical Jargon?

Professionals from any field are known to develop their own language, jargon that they use as a form of shorthand. Unfortunately, most people do not know the jargon and may feel too intimidated to ask for explanations.

Here are some of the more common terms that you and your parents are likely to hear, either in the doctor's office, the community clinic, or the hospital.

Explanation of Common Terms

Activities of Daily Living (ADL)

These are everyday activities that most adults can do independently, including bathing, continence, dressing, eating or feeding oneself, toileting, and transferring or mobility (arising from bed and moving about the home environment). Services that support ADLs are called "personal care services" and are provided by workers such as home health aides, nursing assistants, and personal care aides.

Assessment

For government-funded programs, a professional such as a nurse or social worker completes a standardized assessment to determine eligibility for the variety of home, community and facility-based services.

Confidentiality

The term refers to the obligation of a health professional to treat a patient's information as private. Privacy refers to the right of an individual to decide what personal information can be shared with others. The guidelines for confidentiality are found in the professional's code of ethics and in legislation related to privacy.

Cognitive Impairment

The term, also called "dementia," refers to the inability to think, reason, remember, or perceive. Alzheimer Disease is a major cause of cognitive impairment.

Eligibility

For government-funded programs, eligibility is determined through a professional assessment and may include criteria such as age, medical status, residence requirement (e.g. live in the province for one year), and other criteria unique to each program. For privately-funded programs, the client and/or the provider determine eligibility.

Geriatric Team

A geriatric team is comprised of professionals from a variety of disciplines that work together to meet the special needs of older individuals. The team often includes a physician or geriatrician, nurse, occupational therapist, social worker, physiotherapist, and pharmacist. Other professionals might also be involved.

In-Home Services

Professional and personal care services are provided to individuals living in their own home. This may include private dwellings, apartments, seniors' lodges, and congregate dwellings.

Long-term care

Long-term care refers to the variety of services provided to people who experience prolonged physical illness, disability, or cognitive impairment. The purpose of these services is to help people maintain a level of functioning rather than to correct or cure medical problems. Most commonly, assistance with activities of daily living (ADL) and professional care are included.

Mild cognitive impairment (MCI)

Mild cognitive impairment is a general term used to describe a subtle but measurable memory disorder that is greater than normally expected with aging; however, the afflicted person does not show other symptoms of dementia, such as impaired judgment or reasoning.

Transition Unit

This refers to a unit that may be in a hospital or long-term care setting that is designed to provide intermediary care for patients who have been treated for an acute health problem, but are now stable and might be able to return to the community. The unit focuses on the improvement of function in activities of daily living.

Who are the Members of the Healthcare Team?

It can be helpful to you and your parents to become familiar with the various categories of workers in health care. Here is a brief description of the most common team members:

Caregiver

A caregiver is an individual who takes care of an older person, usually to provide personal and supportive care. The term often refers to a family member or friend. In health care, the caregiver may be known as a care attendant, personal care worker, or personal healthcare worker. The education of this category of worker is not standardized. [See also: Home Health Aide]

Case Manager

A case manager is a professional (often a registered nurse or social worker) who oversees the assessment and planning for care and service for an individual. Case managers work in hospitals and community programs. Some Geriatric Case Managers can be hired privately on a fee-for-service basis.

Companion

A companion is an individual who provides housekeeping, meal preparation, shopping, and transportation as well as social support to an older adult living in the community.

Discharge Planner

A discharge planner is an individual (usually a social worker or registered nurse) who works in a hospital and assists patients to connect to healthcare services in the community following a hospital stay.

Geriatrician

A geriatrician is a physician with specialized training or experience in caring for the special health needs of people over the age of 65. Geriatrics is the branch of medicine that deals with the problems and diseases of old age.

Gerontological Nurse

A gerontological nurse is a registered nurse with specialized knowledge and education in aging. These nurses work with older adults and their families in both hospital and community settings. "Gerontology" is the study of aging.

Home Care Coordinator (Community Care Coordinator)

A home or community care coordinator is a registered nurse, social worker, or physiotherapist who assesses and oversees the home care services that are provided to a client. The coordinator assigns the care to the appropriate member of the team.

Home Health Aide

A home health aide is an individual who provides personal care: bathing, dressing, grooming, assistance with eating. These aides may assist with mobility by helping an elderly individual to walk with assistance or supervision. Some may assist with rehabilitation; for example, helping with range of motion exercises and other exercise programs under the direction of a professional such as a physiotherapist. They may also be called a personal support worker or personal care aide. The education of these workers is not standardized.

Licensed Practical Nurse (LPN)

A licensed practical nurse (also known as registered practical nurse) assesses a patient's condition and reports to a registered nurse or physician. LPNs also administer medications and perform some nursing procedures.

Occupational Therapist

An occupational therapist is a professional trained to work with persons with permanent or temporary impairment in physical or mental functioning (including individuals in all age groups). The aim of occupational therapy is to help the client to perform activities of daily living and to develop the skills to live independent, satisfying and productive lives. Occupational therapists conduct both physical and mental assessments.

Pharmacist

A pharmacist is a health professional trained in the art and science of pharmacy. A pharmacist dispenses a medication based on the prescription from the physician (in some jurisdictions, they have the right to prescribe certain medications). Pharmacists play a vital role in helping older individuals to receive safe and effective drug treatment.

Physiotherapist

A physiotherapist is a health professional trained in the treatment of injuries and physical disabilities. (Note: in Canada the term physiotherapist is used; in the U.S., physical therapy is the parallel term.)

Recreational Therapist

Recreational therapists are also referred to as therapeutic recreation specialists. They use a variety of approaches, including music, arts, dance, and structured activities to improve or maintain emotional, mental and physical well-being.

Registered Nurse (RN)

A registered nurse assesses a patient's condition and makes decisions regarding appropriate nursing interventions. RNs can respond to complex situations and work with physicians to establish an appropriate plan of care and treatment. They also administer medications and monitor responses. RNs work in all healthcare settings. In some jurisdictions, registered nurses can prescribe medications.

Social Worker

A social worker is a health professional who works with people viewed as having special disadvantages (i.e. low income, disabilities, mental illness). Social work focuses on social change, problem solving in human relationships and the empowerment of people to enhance their well-being.

How do we Interact with Health Professionals?

Health professionals are key players in assisting you and your parents. Receiving appropriate diagnosis and treatment can make a significant difference to quality of daily life.

A good primary care physician whom your parent trusts can make a big difference. If you live nearby, getting to know the doctor can be very helpful. If possible, ask if you can accompany your parent when he/she visits the doctor. There are several valid reasons for this request.

- You can provide your personal contact information to the office.

- You can provide what is referred to as "collateral information." You can let the doctor know about your observations, which might assist with accurate diagnosis. For example, you might notice that your mom sometimes appears off balance when she moves suddenly. The doctor may review your mom's medications to see if any are causing this problem.

- You can write down a list of questions that both of you want answered and keep notes in a notebook. In this way, you provide a second "set of ears" to hear what the doctor says and review the information after the visit.

- You can ask the doctor about the things that you might do to help your parent. For example, if your mom is on a special diet, such as salt-restricted for treatment of heart failure, the doctor might have helpful advice.

Each of these is a valid reason for attending a visit. Sometimes, it is tempting to call the doctor and talk about your concerns privately. You can do so, however, only with your parent's permission. The doctor will not reveal private healthcare information to you, because of professional confidentiality, and it is most likely that your phone call will not be kept "secret" – the doctor will tell your parent because of the doctor-patient relationship. Think about this – what if the roles were reversed and your parent called your doctor!

Office visits are brief, and you may find that there is not enough time to address all the concerns in one visit. Healthcare professionals are busy, and sometimes you need to use polite persistence in order to gather information and receive services for your parent. You might need to schedule several visits.

If you live at a distance, try to arrange a visit and schedule appointments to meet the doctor, the home and community care coordinator, and others who are involved in providing care or support to your parent.

How can we Advocate for our Parents?

As your parent needs more assistance, you may find yourself in the new roles of advocate or spokesperson. It is best if one family member acts for your parents; this person will contact the care team and keep the rest of the family informed. Consider obtaining a power of attorney, which gives you the legal authority to make decisions on your parents' behalf when they are no longer able to do so. See Chapter Eight for more information.

Here are some ways that you can be an advocate:

1. Keep in touch with the physician. The doctor is responsible for the medical diagnosis and often knows the overall plan.

2. In the hospital, keep in touch with the discharge planner. This individual communicates with members of the team to determine the plan for discharge (including the services that will be needed at home).

3. In the community, keep in touch with the case manager (might also be called community care coordinator).

4. Start a notebook and keep the names and phone numbers of all the professionals that are involved. Ask them to explain their roles.

5. Negotiate specific times for telephone calls to the health professional. Ask if e-mail correspondence is possible.

6. Be assertive in asking for information. Ask your parent to inform the healthcare providers that they can talk to you (if your parent is willing to do so). Inquire about the limits of confidentiality and privacy. What can a family member be told, according to legislation in that particular province?

Useful Resource

Provincial Privacy Legislation is available from PrivacyInfo.ca

http://www.privacyinfo.ca/legi_prov.php?v=10

Take Action

> Jargon can interfere with communication. Try to learn the most common terms and do not be reluctant to ask for explanations.

> Ask healthcare professionals to explain their roles. You and your parent want to know who is most likely to help you solve specific problems.

> Start a notebook or purchase a guide that helps you to keep track of medical information. For example, you might want to purchase the *Personal Care Binder* available from Caregiver Network Inc. http://www.caregiver.on.ca

> Expect to live on a "roller coaster" and to adapt to frequent changes in the plan as your parent's condition and level of functioning changes.

> Recruit help from family and friends. You will need information and support.

Why Geriatrics and Gerontology Matter

The aging process is complex – and unique to each individual. When older adults experience acute illness, they need – and deserve – specialized care. But who has the expertise to recognize normal aging, identify common diseases of old age, and provide holistic care?

The answer: health professionals who have specialized in Geriatrics or Gerontology. The term "Geriatric" refers to the study, diagnosis and treatment of common diseases associated with aging. The term "Gerontology" is derived from Greek, and means "the study of elders." Gerontology is multidisciplinary and therefore looks at physical, mental, and social aspects of a senior's life.

Why know these terms? Because there are a variety of practitioners in your community, knowing how to find those with specialized knowledge and expertise will help you or a senior family member get the best possible care.

In hospital: A geriatrician is as important to an older adult as a pediatrician is to a child! So ask for a geriatrician – a physician who can work with the healthcare team to determine an appropriate plan of care. Geriatricians have been certified in Canada since 1981.

In a long-term care facility: Ask for a Certified Gerontological Nurse. These nurses have written national certification exams to demonstrate their knowledge and skills. Their education makes them exemplary problem-solvers. As part of the healthcare team, their focus includes avoiding the dangers of over-treating as well as under-treating chronic and acute health problems in older adults.

In the community: If a senior is still healthy and wants to stay that way as long as possible, look for a Geriatric or Gerontological Nurse Practitioner. Contact your local health authority or the provincial nursing association to locate resources near you.

Source: ElderWise Info, V2: No 9 May 2006

Reprinted with permission. www.elderwise.ca

PART 3

PLAN AHEAD

CHAPTER SEVEN

NAVIGATING THE MAZE:

FINDING THE SERVICES

Perhaps you are wondering if Dad is showing signs of memory loss, but you don't know where to go for assessment. Or you find yourself wishing that Mom would to go to a doctor who knows more about aging. You might be looking for in-home services and feel confused when you try to find them. You think that Mom would be much safer if she used a cane or a walker – but where do you buy it, and how can you be sure that it is right for her? How will you accomplish all this if you live at a distance?

Questions answered in this chapter:

How do we know what services we need?
What support can our family provide?
What types of services are available?
What are the differences between public and private services?
Where do we find the services?
How do we influence our parents to accept the services?

How do we Know What Services we Need?

Assessment

Assessment of needs is the first step. Talk to your parents to obtain their perspective on what they need in order to maintain or improve the quality of their daily life. Then ask their permission to meet with their family physician. Tell the doctor that you want to talk about your present and future concerns. Call or visit the nearest seniors' centre; staff may have or know about seniors health programs that offer outreach assessment services. Also find out about "geriatric services" - specialized care for the common illnesses associated with aging. You might find a geriatric care manager or a gerontological nurse practitioner at the local hospital or community clinic.

According to Statistics Canada, the most common services needed by seniors living in the community are

- help with housework and maintenance chores (67%),

- transportation, help with banking and shopping (51%),

- family or friends checking on them by telephone (39%),

- emotional support (23%),

- and personal care assistance (12%).

By about the age of 85, almost half of seniors need some assistance with their activities of daily living. These activities, known by the acronym ADLs, include mobility, bathing/showering, eating, and dressing. Some of these needs can be met by family and friends; others can be met by home or community care and support services.

What Support can our Family Provide?

When you have an assessment that identifies what type of help is needed, it might be a good time to have a family meeting to discuss the needs and decide on an initial plan of action. When arranging for this meeting, have an agenda to help stay on topic and try to make sure that everyone has an opportunity to share his or her thoughts and ideas. You can use the following questions to help frame your family discussion.

- What are your parents' current health problems, including physical and cognitive limitations?

- Are there ways to rearrange or renovate the house for greater independence and safety?

- What services are needed at home?

- What is the financial situation? Can your parent afford to pay for services?

- What exactly needs to be done? What tasks can each member of the family do? (Make a list of assignments.)

- What will each family member do to support the others, particularly the primary caregiver (i.e. the person assigned overall responsibility for coordinating the assistance)?

- What might be needed in the future concerning care, services, housing, transportation, and finances?

- How is everyone feeling about the plan? Are there any fears or emotional issues?

- When will you meet or communicate next?

Create a detailed written plan, including schedules and assignments, and provide a copy for each person.

What Types of Services are Available?

Now that you and your parents have some ideas about their needs, it is helpful to be aware of services that are available for seniors living in the community. These services are provided through both public and private providers (more on the difference between them later in this chapter).

General Types of Public Services

A range of services is offered through the publicly funded healthcare system. The main sectors include adult day care, geriatric assessment, home care, public health, respite, and facility based care. Each of these is summarized below:

Adult day care programs are often operated within a long-term care centre or other health or social facility. Some programs provide social activities while others include medical surveillance and some direct care. Most programs offer regular attendance that varies from two days to five days per week.

Geriatric assessment units admit people for a limited period of time to assess and determine care needs. Many acute care or rehabilitation hospitals have these special short-term units that do a complete assessment of medical and cognitive function. The team often includes nurses, physicians, physiotherapists, occupational therapists, dietitians, social workers, and other specialists. The team consults with the family about recommended services that are available after discharge.

Home care (or community care) programs are managed by local health authorities and vary across the provinces. Home care services include a variety of programs that are offered in the community to help people remain in their own homes, to reduce hospital admissions, and facilitate earlier discharge. For the most part, home care is provided at minimal cost to a client who has a health problem that requires professional support (such as that given by registered nurses, therapists, and social workers) or regular personal care provided by home health aides. The professional acts as a case coordinator and can assist family members with referrals and other related services.

Facility-based care refers to the variety of services provided to people who experience prolonged physical illness, disability, or cognitive impairment. The purpose of these services is to help people to maintain a level of functioning, rather than correct or cure medical problems. Some facilities, such as Assisted Living, provide supportive housing and personal care. (See Chapter Nine for more information on these housing options.) Other facilities provide 24-hour nursing and professional care.

- These facilities have different names across the provinces, such as Nursing Homes, Residential Care Facilities (RCF's), Homes for the Aged, Extended Care, Personal Care Homes, and Long Term Care Centre (LTCC).

- Most provinces provide facility-based care as part of the publicly funded services; however, there are provincial differences. Usually the medical portion of costs is covered while the client is responsible for the accommodation (food and lodging) portion of the costs. For the most part, admission is through a "central assessment" or single point of entry that is administered by local health authorities.

Public health units include teams of community health nurses who focus on health promotion and prevention for well seniors. Programs vary, but many provide routine immunization (e.g. flu shots), public education sessions, falls prevention programs, and group or individual counseling. Community health (or public health) nurses are also knowledgeable about other services.

Respite care is temporary support, given to provide relief to the family. If Mom is taking care of Dad at home and needs a break, you will want to find respite, or relief services. There are three different ways for this service to be provided: in-home care, adult day programs, and short-stay care. In-home care will bring someone into the home of the senior to help with personal care. Adult daycare programs enable the senior to meet other people and enjoy activities away from home. The program may also offer therapeutic activities, meals, transportation to and from the program, and some personal care. Short-stay respite allows a senior temporary access to the care at a long-term care facility.

Community Services
If your parents need the most common types of support identified earlier in the chapter, where will you find these services? There are many services provided by voluntary, not-for-profit and for-profit organizations.

A brief description of the most common services follows.

Banking. To reduce the risk of fraud, you and your parents should talk about reliable help with banking. If you are going to provide this assistance, make an appointment with your parent's personal banker. This individual can help to set up automatic payment systems and suggest other ways to protect against scams.

Counselling. Any time of transition and change can have profound emotional repercussions. For some people, having the help of a professional psychologist, social worker, or family therapist can provide coping strategies, a new outlook, or just a safe place to discuss issues freely. Many religious groups also provide counselling or support groups.

Emergency response systems. For peace of mind, many seniors subscribe to services that will install a system that allows for daily phone contact and emergency notification in case of a fall or illness. Some communities provide programs that monitor the safety and security of a senior who is living alone. Contact your local health authority for more information.

Emotional support. Although you might assume that only family can provide emotional support, this overlooks the value of others. Friends, neighbors, church groups, volunteer organizations, and peer support groups are key players in the provision of emotional support to you and your parent.

Foot care. Foot care services provide help trimming toenails, monitoring the feet for health and changes, and bathing or massaging the feet.

Home maintenance and repair. There are pubic agencies and private companies that provide yard maintenance and snow removal. Some will also clean windows and arrange for repairs that involve plumbing or electrical work. Some agencies will arrange the entire job depending on the health of the senior.

Home support. Workers come to the home to help with activities such as meals, light housekeeping, and laundry. Others will offer transportation to medical appointments.

Meal services. For mobile seniors, some services will provide transportation to a dining hall to join others for a meal. For example, seniors' housing complexes might offer such a program. The advantages include good nutrition and socialization. For those who need to stay at home, services such as "Meals on Wheels" will deliver a meal, and provide some social contact and an informal check as the delivery person will often stay for a brief chat. Also, "Meals on Wheels" will deliver meals at regular intervals rather than everyday, if the senior feels capable of cooking some of his or her meals during a week.

Medication assistance. Talk to a pharmacist about packaging medications in a dosette, or bubble pack. Ask home care agencies if they provide services to assist with medications. If your parent needs reminders, using a daily chart or alarm on a wristwatch may help.

Personal care assistance refers to a range of essential daily activities. Paid caregivers may help with mobility, such as walking or getting into a wheelchair, and with personal care, such as bathing, using a toilet, or dressing. There are many titles given to formal workers who provide such types of care. These may include "Personal Support Worker," "Healthcare Aides," "Personal Care Workers," or "Attendants."

Shopping. Some home support agencies will offer companionship services. Often these companions are individuals with previous experience in providing care to an older person. As a general rule, they do not provide personal care but will offer social visiting, recreational activities, and help with everyday activities such as shopping.

Supplies and equipment. You are probably aware of the usual types of equipment such as canes, walkers, and bathroom grab bars. Visit a home care or a medical supply store in your community, and you will be surprised by the variety of equipment that can make life easier and safer for a frail senior.

Transportation. There are clubs and community based organizations that will help with affordable, reliable, and accessible transportation to activities and appointments. Religious groups and charitable organizations also provide this service. Some public-transit companies provide door-to-door service for wheelchair patrons. Some transit providers allow "stop request" for their senior customers. This allows senior passengers to disembark at a location along the bus route that is closer to their destination even if it is not a bus stop. Some communities have innovative services such as

Driving Miss Daisy. Visit www.drivingmissdaisy.net for more information.

Volunteer services. Canada is a country that supports volunteerism at all ages and stages of life. There are many individuals and organizations that offer support to seniors through the dedicated efforts of volunteers.

What are the Differences between Public and Private Services?

Home and community care services are offered through both public and private providers. Public services are funded and managed by the local health authority. Services are provided on the basis of assessed need. A professional assessment of individual needs, existing supports, and community resources determines eligibility.

There are many private providers offering a variety of home care and support services. Some are non-profit organizations; others are business corporations. These providers vary in types of services, staff qualifications, and costs. It is very common for seniors who want to stay in their home to mix different types of services, both public and private.

Looking for a quality service provider can be challenging. See the checklist at the end of this chapter to help you find the best provider for your parent's needs.

Where do we Find the Services?

There are many services available to seniors in Canada, both in urban and rural areas. It may take some time to sort through what is available and how to access these services.

Begin by asking your parents; they often have a great grapevine through their friends who know the services that are available in their community. Spend the time upfront making calls, talking to agencies and to others who have cared for a relative in your parent's community.

If you live at a distance, you may find the Internet very helpful. A word of advice: you will want to use reliable sites. Read *How to Find Trustworthy Information on the Internet* from the Canadian Health Network at the end of this chapter.

It is also useful to find a significant connection in your parents' community. During one of your visits, get to know your parents' community – from their perspective. Who are their neighbors? Will they respond in time of need, and will they give you their phone number? And before you leave, obtain a copy of the current local telephone book – it might be very useful if you need to find support services in the future.

Useful Resources

If you are looking for services, you can try these sources of information.

General Information for Seniors Services

- Check the local phone book. Most directories have pages dedicated to seniors' services.

- Call the Government of Canada 1-800-O-CANADA (or 1-800-622-6232).

- Visit the website of Seniors Canada On-line: http://www.seniors.gc.ca/index.html

- Call the local health authority.

- Contact local seniors clubs and associations.

Specific Services

- To find assistive devices or equipment (e.g. walker, bath bench, or hospital bed), look for "medical supply" or "homecare stores." Contact the local Red Cross.

- Check with the local health authority.

If you live at a distance and want to find contact information for specific services, try the tips in the box below.

Tips for Finding Services at a Distance

- Consider having the assistance of a Geriatric Care Manager. Visit one of the following websites for more information on the role of these health professionals.
  (1). www.diamondgeriatrics.com
  (2). www.caregiver.on.ca

- Use the Internet. To use the Internet wisely, check out the guidelines from the Canadian Health Network at the end of this chapter.

- Go to www.411.ca

- See "Searching for Services at a Distance" at the end of this chapter.

How do we Influence our Parents to Accept the Services?

You've talked to your mom, and you know that her life would be so much easier – and safer – if she would agree to homemaking services and some personal care assistance. But she refuses. Now what can you do?

First, you know your parent's personality and long time patterns of being independent or accepting help from others. If you have never been able to influence your parent, it is not very likely that you will be able to do so now. You might have to rely on others, such as a sibling, another relative, or a good friend to talk to you parents.

If you think that your parent might be reluctant but receptive, here are a few ways to introduce the idea of using services:

- Purchase help such as yard work, home maintenance or annual cleaning as a gift. You parents may be pleased to try out the service and to accept your good intentions.

- Talk to others for recommendations about services or programs in the local community. Get a list for your parents, with contact names and numbers.

- Arrange for a new service provider to come to the home when you are there. This might alleviate the worry of letting strangers into the house. You can also offer to follow up if the service does not meet expectations.

Take Action

If you and your parent have agreed that more help and support are needed, here are some steps to take:

> Determine the needs for services. First, talk to your mother or father. Offer your own observations. Involve others, such as the doctor or other health professionals to talk about current and future needs.

> Have a family meeting to assess the situation. What are your family's strengths and resources? What are the demands and challenges? Mutually agree on roles and responsibilities.

> Investigate publicly funded services.

> Where necessary and possible, augment with private services.

> Use the Checklist for Private Healthcare Agencies at the end of this chapter to ensure that the service provider is reliable.

How to Find Trustworthy Information on the Internet

About the author
√ Is the author's name included? Is he/she a professional or accredited authority on the subject?
√ Does the author rely on personal experience? For example, he or she is writing about MS and has MS.
√ Does the site provide a phone number or email for the author?

About the organization
√ If an organization is listed as the source of the information, is it recognized as an authority on the subject?
√ Are medical or scientific terms clearly explained?
√ What kind of scientific evidence is provided?

About your privacy
√ Are privacy guidelines clearly stated?
√ If you need to register to use the site, is your privacy ensured?

About the site
√ Is the site user friendly?
√ Is there an email to contact a web manager or administrator if you have problems with the site?
√ Does the site include Canadian content?
√ How current is the information on the site?
√ Is the site trying to sell you something?
√ Does the site offer a clear statement that health information should not be taken as health advice or a substitute for visiting a health professional?
√ If there are fees associated with use of the resources on the site, are they clearly explained?

Adapted from the Canadian Health Network
http://www.canadian-health-network.ca

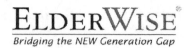

Checklist: Evaluating Private Healthcare Agencies

Accreditation
√   Is the agency accredited? A company that has accreditation
    has been through a recognized evaluation, for example,
    through the Canadian Council on Health Services
    Accreditation.

Suitability
√   Does the provider have the type of service that you require
    now and in the future?
√   Do they offer the service during the hours that you require?
√   Is the waiting period for services acceptable?
√   Are the costs affordable?

Reputation.
√   How do others describe this service provider?

Staff
√   What type of staff does the agency provide? (RN, LPN, Home
    Healthcare Aide, Home Maker, Companion)
√   Are all the staff insured and bonded?
√   Does every staff member undergo a criminal record check?
√   Does the agency attempt to provide consistent staff members?
√   Does the agency have back-up protocol if a staff member fails
    to show for work?

Eligibility requirements.
√   Does the agency provide a professional assessment prior to
    initiating services?
√   Are there criteria that might exclude services?

Searching for Services at a Distance

Your parents live in one province, and you live in another. Your dad has early dementia and lives at home with your mom. You and your siblings have suggested to your mom that you want to find someone to help her with housework and personal care. She agrees – now where do you look?

In addition to using the resources listed in this chapter, you can also find a local home healthcare agency by using one of the following services.

(1) Visit the website of YellowPages.ca
http://www.yellowpages.ca/index.html

You can search by business category or location. For example, you can search for "home healthcare" in your parents' city. A comprehensive list of agencies found in that city will be identified. When the list of agencies appears, you can read about each agency to find out more about their location and their services. For example, you might find one that specializes in providing care and support to individuals with Alzheimer Disease.

(2) Instant messaging (IM). You can use IM on a PC, PDA, or cell phone. If you need instructions for IM, visit the website of illumiCell and download "Quick Start for Yellow Pages IM Search." www.illumicell.com

Using the service of illumiCell allows you to find the agencies that are closest to your parents' home. For example, you can put in your parents' postal code, along with the words "home healthcare" and a list of the nearest agencies will be identified. You can obtain contact information for each agency.

CHAPTER EIGHT

TAKING CARE OF BUSINESS:

FINANCIAL AND LEGAL MATTERS

Aging means change and transition. Change is what happens around you; transition is the journey that you take to manage the change. But not everyone in the family manages change and transition in the same way. How do you react to change? How will your style of coping with change influence the way that you plan for the future? How will it affect other members of your family?

> **Questions answered in this chapter:**
>
> *How can we talk about money, a sensitive and personal subject?*
> *What are the personal costs of aging?*
> *What is available to help with the costs?*
> *What should we know about Elder Law?*

Let's assume that families are made up of "reactors," "actors," and "proactors."

First, let's talk about the REACTORS. These are the people who tend to wait for things to happen and then react. They spring into action and get things done, or they rely on others to help them to manage. They are not likely to worry too much about the future but more likely to live in the present and perhaps hold on to the past. When others tell them that they need to plan, they might reply, "Plan for what? No one has a crystal ball."

You might hear a "reactor" tell others to stop worrying. "Worry," they say, "is like a rocking chair; keeps you busy but gets you nowhere." Reactors have certain beliefs and assumptions that work for them. They believe that, usually, things will work out for the best. They assume that they will receive help if they need it.

Next, there are the ACTORS. These are the people who do some preparation for the future. They learn the script. They know their role. They ask questions and gather information. They know that things change as they grow older, but they do not take steps until they have to.

The "actors" might give the appearance of listening to others, but then may not take action, unless they agree with the advice. Overall, they tend to get things done, by themselves or with others, but just in time.

And then there are PROACTORS. These people look to the future; they are often heard talking about tomorrow, next year. They ask "What IF?" They devote some energy to worrying or at least thinking about possible changes.

"Proactors" prefer to plan ahead as this gives them a sense of control. They value being "proactive"and might voice an opinion that everyone else should be. They want to act before a situation becomes a crisis.

Now think about your family. Do you have "reactors," "actors," and "proactors?" Which term describes you the best? How might these differences help or hinder conversations that your family has about the future?

How can we Talk About Money, a Sensitive and Personal Subject?

What does "money" mean to each generation in your family? Many of today's older adults (for example, those over 75) hold values about money that are different from those of their adult children. Recall the different world views of veterans and boomers explored in Chapter Four.

People born in Canada in the 1930's arrived when the "Great Depression" was influencing everyone's life. Wasting "anything" troubles some of these seniors. One depression-era senior said that when she was growing up, she never remembers seeing a full garbage pail because they used every bit of what ever they had. We tend to think of more recent generations as being the "green generation," but many who lived through and survived the Great Depression were the original reduce, reuse, and recycle generation.

Seniors with this experience may worry about running out of money. They would never use expressions such as "it's only money" or "that's that cost of doing business." And if you say these things, they may feel insulted rather than relieved. They may be willing to go without rather than spend money.

Another group of Canadian seniors were born in Europe and were young children when WWII erupted. They experienced the effects of war and immigration first-hand. For this generation, financial status may relate not only to the amount of money they have, but also to the fear that another event, out of their control, might take it away. They may distrust banks and financial institutions. They may view money as a very private matter, a subject that should remain closed.

In some traditional households, the man handles the financial affairs. The woman, therefore, may not be fully informed of their assets or debts. Some women learn that they are wealthy or poor only when they are widowed! These women might also have to learn new skills of money management at this difficult time.

Tips for Talking About Money

- Try to understand your parents' beliefs and anxieties about money.

- Explain that you want to talk about money not because you want the details, but because you want to know the future possibilities.

- If your widowed mother lived in a traditional marriage and now must handle the finances, try to reassure her that learning a new skill always causes some anxiety. Offer to help her yourself, or if that is uncomfortable, talk to the manager at your mother's bank for advice.

- Talking about money is more than "factual." It is a highly emotional issue. Reassure your parent that you are not judging their handling of money; you are looking to help, and helping requires knowing the full situation. Keep in mind some of the emotional issues mentioned above.

What are the Personal Costs of Aging?

Old age, and its physical, social, psychological, and emotional changes, can be an expensive life stage. Some of the costs are covered or partially covered by public healthcare, depending on provincial funding. Some families are surprised to learn that many costs are not covered.

Partially Covered

- Hearing aids
- Dental care
- Medications
- Home and medical equipment (basic equipment such as canes and walkers)
- Home care (for personal and medical care)

Not Covered

- Home support (companion, meal service, grocery shopping)

- Transportation

- Maintaining an old home

- Assistance with yard work

- Assistance with housework

- Rising taxes

- Retirement housing

What is Available to Help with the Potential Costs of Aging?

This chapter has information about important issues related to planning for the future. Don't feel you have to have a full understanding of all the terms and suggestions made throughout the following pages. The information is designed to introduce you these options and get you thinking about which ones might work for you.

Senior Benefit Programs

There are many seniors benefits programs, both provincial and federal, that are not utilized by those who qualify. Here are a few examples:

- Deferred taxes

- Enhanced healthcare benefits (vision care, dental care)

- Assistance with home renovations

- Assistance with Aids to Daily Living (home and medical equipment, such as walkers and bath chairs.)

Useful Resource

Contact the provincial government for information on benefit programs in that specific province.

Long-Term Care Insurance

In contrast to critical illness insurance, long-term care insurance is intended to help pay the costs associated with long-term care, whether in the home or in a facility. Because there are no standardized policies, you need to become knowledgeable about what is covered and what is exempt.

Useful Resource

J. O'Donnell, G. McWaters, & J. Page have written a helpful reference, *The Canadian Retirement Guide.* You will find several chapters on financial planning.

What Should we Know about Elder Law?

An Elder Law attorney is a lawyer who specializes in issues concerning older adults. Some of the areas addressed in Elder Law are competency or capacity, guardianship, enduring power of attorney, and healthcare directives.

What about Competency?

Competency or capacity refers to the ability to understand and to execute a document. It means being legally qualified to perform an act. It is also defined as the mental ability to distinguish right from wrong and to manage one's own affairs.

Only qualified professionals, such as psychologists, psychiatrists, physicians, and occupational therapists, can determine whether an individual is mentally competent. To be competent, the person must show an ability to understand information in such a way as to make a decision and to realize the likely consequences of the decision. Mental capacity is a complex issue. An individual may be deemed competent to make decisions in some areas and not in others. For example, the person might be able to make healthcare decisions but not decisions involving property.

Competency is not the same as reasonableness or rationality. This is an important distinction. Your parents, just like yourself, can make foolish or unreasonable decisions, but such errors are not sufficient to deem them incompetent!

If your parent is declared mentally incompetent, you can act on his/her behalf if you are named the agent in a healthcare directive. If such a document does not exist, you might have to apply for guardianship and power of attorney, explained below.

What is Guardianship?
Guardianship is a legal process in which an individual is named the guardian of a dependent person and given both the right and the responsibility to act in the other person's best interests.

Each province has provisions to protect the rights of vulnerable individuals. One such protection occurs through the Public Guardian and Trustee. In general terms, a Public Guardian and Trustee manages the affairs of people who do not have healthcare directives in place and do not have an appointed guardian or trustee.

Useful Resource

For more information on laws related to Public Guardian and Trustee contact your provincial government.

What is Power of Attorney?
Power of attorney is the legal authority to make decisions on behalf of those who have lost capacity to make their own decisions. The document applies to each specific province; therefore, you need to consult a lawyer who understands the powers and limitations within that jurisdiction.

What is the value of power of attorney (POA)? Everyone, not just older people, should grant power of attorney to a trusted family member or friend. It allows you to name a person to act for you, in the event that you become mentally incapable, either temporarily or permanently.

What is a Healthcare Directive?

A personal healthcare directive is a written document that provides instructions about medical treatment in the event that an individual cannot express his or her wishes. It includes specific instructions and identifies a proxy or agent who will speak on behalf of the individual. Writing down one's wishes can ease the pressure on family members when they are faced with difficult decisions.

Sometimes a healthcare directive is referred to as a "living will." The actual terms and limits for healthcare directives vary among provinces. What these legal directives have in common is that each enables people to make their own decisions about medical care and treatment and to ensure that others are aware of these personal choices.

You can choose to have a lawyer write the document, or do it yourself as long as you ensure that the document is legal in your province or territory. You should not help your parents to write the document unless you are familiar with the laws within their province.

If you, or your parents, are interested in writing a directive, take these steps.

1. Find out more information that applies to your province.

2. Talk to your family doctor who can help you to make an informed decision.

3. Talk to your family and friends.

4. Write the directive or seek help from a lawyer.

5. Keep a card in your wallet/purse indicating the name of your substitute decision-making (proxy) and the location of the directive.

6. Update the document from time to time. Changes in your health status, as well as advances in medicine, might influence your decisions.

Useful Resources

Federal Government. For information on all federal government programs, call 1-800-667-3355.

Health Canada. http://www.hc-sc.gc.ca

Veterans' Affairs Canada. Call 1-800-387-0919 or visit http://www.vac-acc.gc.ca/general

Take Action

➤ Talking about money is almost always a very sensitive subject.

➤ Be aware that not all services are covered by the publicly-funded healthcare system. Become familiar with benefit programs offered by provincial and federal governments.

➤ Make it a priority to write your health and personal care directive! Encourage your parents to do the same. Keep copies of your directive and your parents' directives if you are named their agent or proxy.

➤ If you named an agent for your parent, you may have to make tough decisions. Consult others. Seek support.

CHAPTER NINE

THE MEANING OF HOME

When you hear the word "home" what do you think? A home is a private domestic sphere that forms part of a person's identity. The family home also serves an important role for the extended family. More commonly we think about the following:

- Home is where the heart is

- There's no place like home

- Home is an environment that offers affection and security.

Questions answered in this chapter:

Where do seniors live? How can we talk about moving?
How can we help our parents to remain at home?
How can we help our parents to move?

A home is

".. largely symbolic .. a place for harbouring the memories, traditions, and personal history of the family. It can act like a living museum, indelibly preserving the various aspects of a family's life cycle ... familiar things .. that engender a special time.. or offering a sanctuary from the demanding world in which we live" (Ralph Hubele, 2004).

Where do Seniors Live?

Canadian Seniors Own Their Own Homes
According to the Canadian Division of Aging and Seniors, a substantial majority of seniors own their home. Most older adults say that they want to continue living in their home as long as possible.

Seniors Live in Urban and Rural Areas
The large majority of Canadian seniors live in an area classified as urban. Seniors, however, are more likely than younger people to live in a rural area: 24% versus 21%. Seniors are also more likely to reside in smaller urban areas.

Seniors Live Alone and With Families
According to the National Advisory Council on Aging, the majority of seniors live in private households, and more than one-half live with a spouse. About 30% live alone, and this includes individuals who are widowed as well as those who are single. Only 7% live with members of their extended family, a number that has steadily declined over the past two decades. There are many reasons why fewer seniors live with the extended families, such as increasing mobility of the younger generation and changes in family structures due to divorce, remarriage, and blended families.

Some Seniors Live in Long-term Care Facilities
The National Advisory Council on Aging tell us that approximately 10% of all people over the age of 65 years live in an institution, and that the proportion of seniors living in these facilities has been declining. These seniors require professional care on a constant basis.

How can we Talk About Moving?

Like many subjects in this book, the topic of housing can be very personal and sensitive. "I am not moving: you will take me out of here feet first." How many times have we heard an older person make this declaration? And indeed, many seniors can remain in their homes into old age. As a result of the physical changes that occur with aging, some individuals prefer to move from their home, and others find it necessary to do so. Having a conversation with your parents whether to "stay put" or "move on" can make a difference between moving by choice and moving out of necessity. Moving by choice usually occurs because the person wants to be closer to family or does not want the burden of household and yard maintenance. The parent may wisely decide to move to a safer environment or to one that provides socialization and personal support. Sometimes illness, accident, or disability dictates the necessity to move from independent living into a facility that provides personal or medical care and services. It is wise to think about options before a crisis occurs, for it is better to choose to move rather than be forced to do so.

Benefits of "moves of choice"	Reasons why "moves of necessity" may occur
• Choice of timing	• Illness, disability
• Choice of location	• Widowhood
• Planned downsizing	• Losses (e.g. driving, income)
• Family decision	• Excessive home maintenance

Want to have a discussion about moving?

- Ask your parent – "If you had to move, what would you miss the most about your current living environment?"

- Make a list of what both you and your parent want and need. Explore why your family wants these things and what you will do if some are not available.

- You might need to have this conversation several times. Try to be patient – although you might already have decided that moving is the best solution, your parent might have been thinking about ways to stay put.

What is a Livable Community?

The surrounding community is as important as the actual home. According to an AARP report, the qualities of a "livable community" include

- Social recreation centres for seniors
- Convenient meeting places
- Volunteer opportunities
- Dependable public transportation
- Safe walking (i.e. well-designed sidewalks)
- Road designed for safe driving (i.e. well-marked signs)
- Security and safety
- Affordable housing options (alternatives to private homes)
- Accessible home (private home)

Your parents can take an interactive quiz on the AARP website to assess their community. See the useful resource on the following page.

Useful Resource

Beyond 50.05 A Report to the Nation on Livable
Communities: Creating Environments for Successful Aging
Research Report. May 2005. A. Kochera, A. Straight, & T.
Guterbock. Available from the website of AARP.
http://www.aarp.org

Full link http://www.aarp.org/research/housing-
mobility/indliving/beyond_50_communities.html

How can we Help our Parents Remain at Home?

Like many seniors, your parents may prefer to remain
in their home, a place that is familiar and gives a sense of
personal control. You might be happy that the family home
remains intact, providing a link to the past. But you might
also worry about safety and the ongoing demands of home
maintenance.

Both generations are concerned about safety. The
Home Safety Council provides tips to prevent dangers and a
list of actions that can secure the home.

- Keep emergency contact numbers by the phone. Include
home phone and address because it is easy to forget this
in an emergency situation.

- "Fall proof "the home – remove scatter rugs, clutter, add
handrails and nightlights, encourage proper footwear.

- Put a temperature limit on the hot water taps.

- Eliminate fire hazards.

- Install an emergency response system.

Making the Decision

Use the checklist on the following pages to determine whether staying in the home is the best option for your family. As you explore each area you might identify barriers to remaining in the home. Remember to be creative and explore community resources. As Alex Mihailidis writes in the Seniors Housing Update (11-2-2002),

> We are beginning to see significant increase in the development of technology-based devices and environments to assist and care for older adults. New innovations such as advanced mobility aids, automatic reminding systems and smart homes have started to emerge with the goals of helping people perform activities independently, and remaining in their own homes for as long as possible.

Although much research and development needs to be done, this emerging field will influence the choice of housing options for older people.

On the next pages, you will find a checklist that you and your parents can use to determine the suitability of staying in the home. You can copy this checklist and have a conversation with your family.

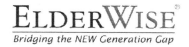

Bridging the NEW Generation Gap

Checklist: Staying at Home

Is your home suitable and safe?
√   How difficult is it for you to manage the stairs in your home?
√   How willing or able are you to clean your home?
√   How willing or able are you to maintain the yard and outside of the home?
√   Do you have enough help available when necessary; e.g. during a short-term illness?
√   Are you at risk for falls? Does your home have good lighting, bathroom safety bars, handrails, and safe flooring?
√   Do you smoke? Do you have and maintain enough smoke detectors?
√   Do you have an emergency response system in case of illness or injury?

Is the choice to stay in your home economically sound?
√   Are taxes, insurance, utilities, and other costs affordable for you?
√   What minor and major repairs must you make in the next few years?
√   Can you get financial assistance for renovations or adaptations?
√   Would freeing up the cash in your home allow you to have a more enjoyable lifestyle?

Is the location of your home suitable?
√   Is adequate transportation available for medical appointments, social activities, and visiting friends and family?
√   Are stores and other services within easy reach?
√   Is the neighbourhood safe and pleasing to you?
√   Do you value the relationships you have with your neighbours?

√   Do you have adequate access to friends, social and church activities?
√   Is your own physical mobility or driving ability an issue?

Are necessary in-home support services available and/or affordable for you?

Do you need the following services? Can you find them and afford them?

√   Household services (cleaning, yard work, minor repairs.)
√   Home-delivered meals. Grocery delivery.
√   Visitors, companions, drivers, etc. – volunteer or paid.
√   Access to adult day programs (if required).
√   Personal care services.
√   Professional services (physiotherapy, nursing).

<u>After completing the checklist and talking about your responses, how would you answer the following question?</u>

Is the decision to stay at home in the best interests of all of your family?

☐ Definitely yes   ☐ Maybe   ☐ Definitely not

How can we Help our Parents to Move?

Even before the decision to move is made, you can suggest that it is a good idea to start looking at housing options. Begin by finding out what is available in your parent's community.

What Housing Options are Available?

There are four main categories of housing, although not every community will have all of these options. The four main categories are

Independent living: housing for those who are functionally independent; includes private single-family dwellings as well as various arrangements of congregate living (e.g.,apartments, condos).

Supportive housing: congregate housing that provides private suites with various types of support for daily but living without medical or professional support.

Assisted living: housing designed to provide both accommodation and personal care.

Long-term care: public and private facilities that provide professional support (nursing, medical, therapeutic) twenty-four hours a day.

Independent Living

Accessory apartment refers to a self-contained unit within a residential home. It may also be known as the "Granny Flat." a self-contained unit on the property of the son or daughter. These flats offer the advantages of proximity and privacy.

Another option is to add an apartment to the parent's home for renters, who can help financially or contribute to household chores and maintenance. Costs for renovations are one disadvantage. You also need to think ahead; your parent's physical needs may become too great to be supported in this environment. Before you pick up the hammer, check local building restrictions and explore the financial implications, including insurance and taxes.

Personal or private care home is a privately operated residential home that provides board and personal support. The operator may live in the same home or hire staff that is on-site 24 hours/day. These homes are usually small; for example, there may be between one and six individuals living under the same roof. The emphasis is on normal daily living rather than healthcare. As with other housing options, whether the individual can remain when health needs change varies among the homes. You are wise to ask about the usual length of stay of tenants and the common reasons people have for moving out.

Supportive Housing

Senior citizen lodge or seniors self-contained housing refer to publicly-funded lodges that provide accommodation, meals, housekeeping, and social activities. Most provinces provide an affordable option for low-income seniors. The costs and eligibility criteria differ between the provinces, and even among the different lodges.

Life lease includes apartments or condominiums that offer the right to occupy the dwelling, without the right to purchase. The individual pays an initial sum, as well as on-going maintenance fees. Usually, the tenants do not have a voice in the policies or management of the facility. The name implies that the right to live there would continue throughout the individual's life; however, this may not be accurate, as the person may have to move if more care and support are required because of physical or mental health changes. Each life lease contract is unique. You will need to read the contract very carefully and to seek professional advice before purchasing.

Assisted Living

These residences combine housing, meals, and supportive services such as housekeeping and recreational activities. Most offer transportation for shopping, outings, and medical appointments. Some also provide personal care assistance, such as bathing and dressing and assistance with routine medications. They are available as rental, life-lease, or ownership. Some provinces provide "designated assisted living" in which the resident pays the accommodation charges, and the health authority pays for the personal care and support services.

There is considerable variation in the services, philosophy, and staffing; therefore, the ability of the resident to remain in the setting, as his or her physical and emotional needs change will depend on the philosophy of the owner/operator. Cost is another important factor. Many of the developments are beyond the affordability for low-to-modest income seniors.

You and your parent will need to visit local residences and ask a few vital questions. Talk to residents and family members about their experiences.   If possible, arrange for a short-term stay.   Nutrition is an important factor for physical health, and social meal times can contribute to emotional health. When you visit assisted or supportive housing facilities, have lunch to get the feeling of the atmosphere and culture. Ask about the menu. How often is it changed? What choices are available? Who ensures that the meals and snacks are nutritious? Use the checklist at the end of this chapter.

Should Dad/Mom Move Closer to Their Children?

This might appear to be the best option because it alleviates your worries, brings your parent closer for physical and social support, and may re-unite your extended family. It is a major decision for your parent and is particularly difficult if not done willingly. So – as with other important decisions – talk before you pack.

Here are some topics for that conversation:

- Your parents may have lifelong friends that they enjoy. How will they keep in touch or develop new friends?

- Although you will offer regular support, this may not be as emotionally satisfying as the previous social circle of friends, and familiar patterns of activity.   What do each of you expect from the other regarding social contact?

- In their familiar environment, they may be able to drive a car, something they might lose if they move to a new city. How will they feel about that?

- How will they get around for medical appointments?

- How will they find and join social activities?

Just for a moment, imagine yourself 20 –30 years from now. Are you living in your current home or have you moved to a nicer climate and developed a new social network?   What role do your children play in your daily life? Would you want to uproot and move to an unfamiliar city at the behest of your adult children?

Should Dad/Mom Move in With Your Family?

According to Statistics Canada for the Division of Aging and Seniors, almost a quarter of a million seniors in Canada live with the extended family, and this is more likely to occur with those over 85 years of age. Here is a common scenario that often precedes the event of Mom or Dad moving to live with an adult child. One parent dies, and the other has health problems that cause concern, or is left in a home that is too large. To overcome the worry, the adult child extends the offer for the parent to live with his/her family. Many families think that this will be a temporary arrangement, and then discover that many years go by. The situation becomes more complex and more challenging. So, like any move, it is wise to talk about this before making the decision. Involve everyone: your parent, your spouse, your children, and the extended family, if appropriate.

Think about having a trial run. Invite your parent to stay for a few weeks, and test whether the decision will work for everyone.

If your family is thinking about this option, reflect on the following:

- Is the physical space in your home appropriate and safe?

- Do you have the supportive equipment such as safety rails in the bathroom?

- What is the quality of the relationship between yourself and your parent and between your parent and your children?

- What happens to your lifestyle if your parent moves in? Do you become housebound? Do your children stop inviting friends over? And – who controls the TV?

- How does this new arrangement affect your health? Do you feel better and less stressed? Or are you exhausted and feel like you are walking on eggshells?

And don't forget to try out some "rules of the pool" at the same time. For example, what household tasks will your parent take on? What role will he/she have in family life, particularly with decisions involving your children? Establish open communication. Does your parent feel like a contributing member or a guest? Remember -home is more than where you are – it is where you have the right to be!

Support Before, During, and After the Move

The decision is made, and a new journey begins. Moving is stressful to people of all ages and more so for an older individual who may have reduced energy or difficulty with hearing or vision. This is a time when youthful energy, strong backs, and great patience are needed.

Here are some steps to help make the process go smoothly.

One: If possible, use professional movers. Save your back and the risk of damaging valued possessions. Ask the moving company for information – many have pamphlets that provide useful tips and to-do lists such as change of address, notification to banks, and canceling services.

Two: Explore available supports. Some cities have services that assist seniors to pack, move, unpack, and get settled in.

Three: Plan to downsize. If your parent is downsizing and needs to make decisions about extra furniture and household equipment, hold a family reunion, and let relatives show their interest in the piano or the sofa. Don't forget the grandchildren – they might cherish something that you would overlook. For relatives at a distance, use photographs or e-mail, and get family members talking about things that have significance to them.

These ideas work well in families with open communication patterns, but could cause distress for those that do not get along well. It might be necessary to remind your mother gently that, although the old dresser has great value to her, it does not fit into the homes of her children or grandchildren. You might want to suggest an auction, a yard sale, or donations to a local charity.

Four: Book time beyond moving day to help your parent to adjust and settle in. If the move is into an assisted living facility, ask if a guest room is available. Stay for a day or two, and accompany Mom or Dad into the dining room. You get to sample the food and meet the staff.

Five: Buy a map and get to know the surrounding community. Take a walking tour to find the location of the nearest bank, dentist, barber or hairdresser, church, medical clinic, pharmacy, and grocery store. Drive or take the bus with your parent to become acquainted with the area.

Six: As soon as you leave, send a note or card. When your mom opens her mailbox for the first time, you don't want it to be empty! Ask others to send mail as well, especially for the first month.

Seven: Help with change of address notification! It is a big task to do alone. And you can use the opportunity to review your parent's list of friends and businesses.

Eight: Watch for relocation stress. If Dad seems to be very tired, forgetful, or irritable, and has several complaints about the new home, ask yourself whether he is feeling depressed. Is he sleeping? Has he seen a doctor? Is he feeling lonely? It is possible to be alone in a crowd!

Take Action

➢ Home is more than a building. Home is a place of safety and belonging. When talking to your parents about moving, remember to think about their feelings and their fears.

➢ Today there are more housing options for seniors. This means that you and your parents might need to do some research to find the most suitable option.

➢ Talk before you pack. Have an open conversation about the options. Involve all of the family.

➢ If choosing assisted living, use the checklist at the end of this chapter.

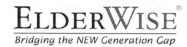

ELDERWISE
Bridging the NEW Generation Gap

Checklist: Assisted Living

Accreditation
√ Is the facility accredited? A company that has accreditation has been through a recognized evaluation process, for example through the Canadian Council on Health Services Accreditation (CCHSA).

Operator's Philosophy and Policies
√ What is the operator's experience in providing services to seniors?
√ Does the operator offer flexibility in the delivery of services?
√ Can the resident choose own physician and pharmacist?

Location
√ Is it easy for family and friends to come to the facility?
√ Are there stores and services within walking distance?

Financial Considerations
√ Is the facility affordable?
√ What are the policies for rent or fee increases?
√ Are there fees for extra services?

Services
√ Do the basic services meet your parent's needs now, and in the future?
√ Are specialty services available (e.g. special diets)?
√ Are the social and recreational programs of interest to your parent?
√ Is transportation provided to medical appointments, and for shopping?
√ What services are available for family and friends (e.g. guest room, meals in dining room)?
√ Is a trial period available?

Environment
√   What is the age and upkeep of the building?
√   Is there an emergency response system?
√   Is there easy access to outdoor space?

Staff
√   What type of staff does the facility provide?
√   Does the staff have recognized qualifications?
√   Are all the staff insured and bonded?
√   Does every staff member undergo a criminal record check?
√   What hours are staff available in the building?

Standards
√   Are there regulatory standards that must be followed?
√   Is there a process for the management of complaints?

Eligibility requirements.
√   Does the agency provide a professional assessment prior to admission?
√   Are there criteria that might exclude admission, or result in moving from the facility?

PART 4

MANAGE

HEALTH CONCERNS

CHAPTER TEN

CHRONIC ILLNESS:

A REALITY FOR SENIORS

At some point, you may be expected to assist your parents in meeting some of their health related needs. How do you feel about that? Does the thought of providing this help make you feel uneasy, or overwhelmed? Do you have sufficient information to provide assistance?

This chapter provides information on the health problems frequently found in seniors and suggests practical ways that you can offer support.

Questions answered in this chapter:

What are the common physical health problems?
> *Hypertension*
> *Heart Disease*
> *Arthritis*
> *Diabetes*
> *Respiratory Disease*
> *Parkinson's*
How can older adults manage chronic illness?
What can I do to provide support?

What are the Common Chronic Health Problems?

The majority of older adults have one or more chronic illnesses. With the correct treatment, some of these illnesses remain stable over a long period of time, while others, such as Parkinson's Disease, are progressive. The majority of individuals can maintain a good quality of life and daily functioning even with chronic illnesses.

Among the most common chronic illnesses are high blood pressure (or hypertension), heart disease, arthritis, and osteoporosis. Other chronic health problems are diabetes, respiratory conditions, and Parkinson's Disease.

About one-quarter of older adults report chronic pain, a condition much more frequently present in those 85+ than in younger people. Pain may limit participation in certain activities and result in regular use of medication, which may increase the risk for injury.

The Challenges of Chronic Illness

Active treatment and management of health concerns should not be discounted in older adults simply because they are "old." Many chronic conditions can be effectively managed to promote optimum health and to avoid the unnecessary complications that may limit activities of daily living. Education is an important aspect of managing chronic illness. If you and your parents understand the symptoms and progression of a chronic condition, it will be easier to face the challenges of the ongoing, ever-present impact of the disease and maximize quality of life.

Hypertension (High Blood Pressure or BP)

Hypertension, or high blood pressure, is the most prevalent cardiovascular disease. As many as 5 million Canadians have high blood pressure and approximately 40% are not aware that they have the condition.

Normal blood pressure, or BP, is measured in

millimeters of mercury and is stated as one number over another.   The   normal   range   of   BP   for   adults   is approximately 120/80. The first number is the pressure exerted by blood on the vessels during the contraction of the heart (systolic), and the second number is the pressure of the blood when the heart is at rest (diastolic). One way to remember the two pressures is that systolic is "squishing" when the heart pushes blood out, and diastolic is "filling" when the heart muscles relax to let blood in.

High blood pressure occurs when the arteries become clogged with fatty deposits (plaque), a condition known as atherosclerosis or arteriosclerosis.

Many factors contribute to high blood pressure; some, such as age and family history are uncontrollable. Others, including obesity, smoking, and stress can be controlled. Regular monitoring is important because hypertension can cause heart attacks, heart failure, stroke, kidney failure, and peripheral artery disease.

Treatment

Treatment consists of managing weight, reducing salt in the diet, limiting caffeine and alcohol, quitting smoking, and using relaxation techniques such as meditation and yoga. Medication may be prescribed to help control blood pressure.

If your parent has hypertension

- High blood pressure is not a normal part of aging. It is the result of hereditary risks and lifestyle.

- Many people with high BP experience no symptoms, so regular measurement is recommended. You can buy equipment and learn to take the pressure or visit a local pharmacy for measurement with a machine. Encourage your parent to keep a record to take to the physician on regular visits.

- Blood pressure can be lowered by diet, weight control, and exercise, but it is not easy to change these aspects of life. Encourage your parent and remember that it is never too late to benefit from lifestyle changes.

- Older people who take medication for high BP may have postural hypotension, a sudden drop in blood pressure when changing from lying to standing position. Here is some advice to prevent fainting. Take these simple steps before standing up: sit on the edge of the bed, then wiggle the toes and dangle the feet for a few minutes.

Useful Resource
The Canadian Hypertension Society has a very useful web site with easy-to- read material. www.hypertension.ca

Heart Disease

Heart disease includes sudden heart attack, chronic congestive heart failure, and irregular heart rhythm. Heart attack is discussed in Chapter Twelve. The problems of congestive heart failure and irregular heart rhythm are described below.

Congestive Heart Failure

When the heart muscle is damaged, the heart is unable to pump blood efficiently. The circulation is impaired, and congestion occurs in the lungs or in the veins in the body. Common symptoms include shortness of breath, fatigue, and swelling in the ankles.

Treatment
For many people with congestive heart failure, medications that strengthen the heartbeat can be very helpful. Diuretics, also known as "water pills," can also be useful. These drugs reduce excess fluid in the body. A lifestyle that balances activity and rest is wise. Limiting salt intake in the diet may be useful. Consult your physician.

If your parent has congestive heart failure

- Lifestyle can reduce the symptoms of congestive heart failure.

- Get adequate rest during the day. Your parent may want to take rest periods after activity.

- Change position. Raise the feet and legs when swelling occurs in the ankles.

- Conserve energy. Learn ways to help your parent conserve energy. For example, if out shopping, take frequent rest stops. If walking, limit or avoid stairs or inclines.

- Use medications carefully. Note that while heart medications and diuretics can be very helpful, these drugs also have side effects. Talk to your parent about ways to take these drugs safely. These drugs should be taken exactly as ordered and at the same time each day. Never double a dose because the drugs can cause toxicity – an adverse effect when the drug level is too high. Refer to Chapter Three for more ideas.

Useful Resource

Read the module *Managing Congestive Heart Failure* developed by The Heart and Stroke Foundation. http://ww2.heartandstroke.ca/images/English/Managing_CHF.pdf

Irregular Heart Rhythm

The normal heart beats 60 to 100 times per minute in response to demand from the body. Specialized cells that conduct electrical currents in the heart control the rhythm and rate of the heart. Many older individuals develop slow heartbeats that can be treated with a small battery-operated device called a pacemaker.

If your parent has a pacemaker

- Pacemakers are inserted in day surgery. The individual may need emotional support prior to surgery and physical support after insertion. For example, for a month following the procedure the person should not do any heavy lifting, extreme stretching, or bending.

- Regular pacemaker check-ups are necessary. This might be done in person at a clinic or through telephone monitoring.

- Your parent should carry a pacemaker ID card to inform healthcare personnel before certain diagnostic tests and in emergencies.

- Remind your parent to tell the dentist. Some electrical equipment should not be used.

- If you are traveling by air, inform security. It might be advisable to avoid the metal detector.

Useful Resource

The Heart and Stroke Foundation. ww2.heartandstroke.ca

Arthritis

Arthritis comprises more than 100 rheumatic diseases. Osteoarthritis is a degenerative joint disease affecting the cartilage of weight-bearing joints. It is the most common form of arthritis and a leading cause of disability and pain in the elderly.

Wear and tear from occupational and recreational activities contributes to osteoarthritis, as do heredity and obesity. Most often the hips, the knees, the lumbar spine, and the neck are affected.

Treatment

Treatment includes rehabilitation, anti-inflammatory medication, and joint replacement surgery. A balance of rest and exercise is recommended.

If your parent has arthritis

- There are specialty medical supply shops across the country with many tools to help people with limited grip and joint stiffness. One example is elastic laces for shoes. These allow the person simply to use the stretch of the elastic to pull the tongue away from the shoe and slide the foot in.

- Tools to help with buttons are also available.

- Check with your parent's doctor. Sometimes physical therapy can be helpful. Heat/cold, massage, and splints are useful to reduce pain and increase mobility.

Useful Resource

The Canadian Arthritis Society. www.arthritis.ca

Osteoporosis

According to the Osteoporosis Society of Canada, as many as 1.4 million Canadians suffer from osteoporosis. As many as one in four women and one in eight men over the age of 50 have the disease.

Osteoporosis is the decrease in the bone mass and density of the skeleton. The bones become more fragile with increased risk for fracture, particularly of the hip, wrist, and spine. Some people have no symptoms. Others may experience a rounding of the back between shoulder blades, called kyphosis. Some may have spinal pain.

Hip fractures are the most serious consequence of this disease. Up to 20% die from complications and as many as 50% are left with some disability after a hip fracture.

Bone loss can be caused by inadequate calcium intake, excessive calcium loss, or poor calcium absorption. Reduced estrogen or androgen (sex hormones), diet, and medications can be factors.

Treatment

Treatment of osteoporosis may include Vitamin D, calcium supplements, hormone therapy, and a diet rich in protein and calcium. Because of the serious consequences of osteoporosis, research is being done to find better prevention and treatment.

If your parent has osteoporosis

- Women are advised to have bone density tests performed regularly for early detection.

- Physical therapy can help. Check with your parent's doctor.

- Activity is important before and after osteoporosis has started. Encourage walking and limited weight bearing exercises as tolerated.

- Many seniors' clubs and assisted living facilities offer fitness or exercise classes, both to residents and to community seniors. Encourage your parent to check into the possibility of joining a program that is specifically designed for older adults.

Useful Resource

Osteoporosis Canada. http://www.osteoporosis.ca

Diabetes

More than two million Canadians have diabetes, a chronic condition with impaired production or release of insulin. Body tissues cannot use glucose, which is needed to fuel the body's cells. Glucose thus accumulates in the blood (hyperglycemia), and this is a serious problem if it persists.

Type 1 diabetes is an absolute lack of insulin and usually begins in childhood or young adulthood.

Type 2 diabetes is much more common and is an inability of the tissues to use insulin as well as a relative lack of available insulin. This type of diabetes usually develops in mid to later life and is increasing in epidemic proportions.

There are serious complications of high blood glucose including: the inability of the body to fight infection, and increased risk of heart disease, blindness, nerve damage, and kidney disease.

As with other diseases, some risk factors are controllable while others are not. Being over 40 and family history are not controllable. Being overweight, on the other hand, can be controlled by diet and exercise. A major risk is fat that accumulates around the midsection. People often refer to this fat deposit as a "spare tire."

Treatment

Treatment for type 1 diabetes includes daily insulin shots, daily blood glucose monitoring, diet for control of glucose levels and weight, physical activity, smoking cessation, managing high blood pressure, and foot care.

Treatment for type 2 diabetes depends on the degree of control over blood glucose levels and may include some or all of the following: daily insulin shots or pills, blood glucose monitoring, diet for control of blood glucose levels and weight, physical activity, smoking cessation, managing high blood pressure, and foot care.

If your parent has diabetes

You can encourage your parent to

- choose footwear that fits very well because wounds on the foot may not heal.

- seek professional foot care,

- travel with candy or juice in case of low blood sugar,

- and have the necessary supplies to check blood sugar.

You can also take the following actions.

- If you are taking your parent to the lab, be certain to inform staff that he/she is a diabetic.

- Notice irritability or sudden mood changes; these can be linked to blood sugar levels, and not just someone being "cranky."

- Learn more about the disease. Find a local Diabetes Association or check out the Useful Resource below.

Useful Resource

The Canadian Diabetes Association. www.diabetes.ca

Respiratory Conditions

Healthy lungs are vital to maintaining a full and active life. Seniors are at high risk for developing respiratory disorders. Smoking and immobility are key factors that contribute to respiratory problems. A number of chronic lung diseases are grouped together and known as chronic obstructive pulmonary disease (COPD). Usually asthma, chronic bronchitis, and emphysema are included.

Asthma

Asthma is a condition where breathing is impaired due to inflammation and constriction in the bronchial tubes of the lungs. Asthma can develop at any age. When a senior has asthma, there is added concern because in older adults this disease places additional strain on the heart. Symptoms include wheeziness, breathlessness, chest tightness, and a cough (often worse at night and early morning).

For some sufferers, the trigger for an asthma attack is an irritant or an allergy. For these people, exposure to pollen, tree fluff, pet dander, or perfume may lead to an attack. Some asthmatics find that their attacks occur after exercise or exertion. Asthma can also be triggered by a viral infection, cold air, or emotional upset.

Treatment

Asthma attacks can have a wide range of severity. Some are more frustrating than dangerous. Each severe attack, however, causes damage to the lungs and needs to be treated. Attacks can also escalate; they can seem mild to start with and then progress, so don't disregard a mild attack. For some asthmatics, attacks are so severe that they stop breathing completely as the bronchial tubes swell shut. This can lead to damage to the brain and the heart. Treatment includes preventing exposure to irritants, relaxation to control breathing, and medications to open the airway and reduce inflammation in the lungs. Individuals with severe attacks often carry an emergency injection of epinephrine, called an "EpiPen."

If your parent has asthma

- Be aware of your parent's allergies, and try to help him or her to avoid these triggers.

- If exercise is a trigger, talk about slowly building up tolerance to exercise.

- When traveling with your parent, be certain that he or she always has the inhaler, even for a short trip to the store.

- If an "EpiPen" is required, be certain it is with your parent at all times. Learn how to give the injection, in case your parent is unable to.

- If an attack is severe or worsens over a short period of time, take your parent for medical attention immediately.

Bronchitis and Emphysema

Chronic bronchitis is common in elderly people. Signs include a persistent, productive cough, wheezing, recurring infections, and shortness of breath. The symptoms may develop gradually, but infections usually become more frequent and difficult to manage. As infection blocks the lungs, people with chronic bronchitis exhale less of the carbon dioxide in their lungs. This means their ability to draw in oxygen is decreased; therefore, less oxygen reaches the tissues. Treatment is aimed at clearing bronchial secretions (mucous) and preventing obstruction of the airway.

Emphysema is a progressive disease caused by changes in the air sacs in the lungs. Causes include chronic bronchitis and chronic irritation from dusts or air pollutants. Cigarette smoking plays a major role in this disease. Onset is slow with gradually more difficulty breathing. Fatigue, poor appetite, weight loss, and weakness are experienced. Recurring chest infections, malnutrition, and congestive heart failure are life-threatening complications of emphysema.

Treatment

Treatment usually includes special physical therapy, medication to open the bronchial tubes, avoiding stress, and breathing exercises. Some individuals require oxygen to ease their breathing.

People with emphysema need a lot of education and support to manage this disease, which requires life style adjustments such as pacing activities, avoiding cold weather, and using the correct medications.

If your parent has lung disease

- At your home, provide a chair with a high back. Your parent might breathe easier when sitting upright.

- When planning outings, be aware of the number of stairs that your parent needs to climb.

- Encourage your parent to learn to avoid exposure to cold weather, to pace activities to conserve energy, and to master deep-breathing techniques.

- If your parent uses oxygen, ask the supplier to teach you and your family about safety precautions.

Useful Resource

Learn more about lung disease. Visit the website of the Canadian Lung Association. www.lung.ca

Parkinson's disease

Many people have an image of a person with Parkinson's, trembling in the hands or legs and twitching of his or her head. Parkinson's is a complicated brain disease in which the receptors in the brain that receive dopamine, a neurotransmitter, begin to die off. Parkinson's disease often begins slowly with tremors of one hand, arm, or leg; these tremors are worse when the limb is at rest. The tremor ceases when the limb is used. The disease progresses to both sides of the body with muscle stiffness, weakness, shuffling walk, stooped posture, and a fixed expression of the face. Further symptoms associated with the disease are shaking of the head, oily scalp and face, depression and anxiety, and difficulty swallowing. In the late stages, loss of mental function may occur. The cause of this disease is unknown.

Treatment

Current treatment for Parkinson's includes drug therapy to reduce the tremors, physical therapy, and speech therapy. There are experimental surgeries, including deep brain stimulation.

If your parent has Parkinson's Disease

- Depression can be part of the disease because of changes in the balance of chemicals in the brain that control mood. Watch for signs and encourage treatment.

- Because the disease affects gait and balance, falls are a risk. Learn more about fall prevention in Chapter Twelve.

- Learn more about the disease. Visit a local chapter of the Parkinson's Society.

Useful Resource

Parkinson's Society Canada. http://www.parkinson.ca

How can Older Adults Manage Chronic Pain?

There is a misperception that pain is a normal aspect of aging. This is not the case. Older people, however, are more likely to have physical conditions that result in both acute, and persistent pain. Pain is an unpleasant subjective experience – there are very few ways to measure pain other than asking the sufferer to try to describe and rate it. Acute pain, generally caused by injury or surgery, usually resolves with healing, and lasts from three to six months. Chronic pain lasts longer than six months, and often results from conditions such as osteoarthritis.

Unrelieved acute pain can be life threatening in older adults because of the increased demand on the heart and other body systems. The social and behavioural effects of chronic pain can have serious impact as well. Frequent assessment and follow-up with healthcare professionals for pain control are important.

Treatment

Treatment using medication can be safe in older people even though they are more susceptible to drug reactions than are younger individuals. The most commonly prescribed drugs are called non-steroidal anti-inflammatory drugs or NSAIDS. Aspirin is one example. Other treatments include massage, heat, cold, and transcutaneous electrical nerve stimulation (TENS). Relaxation (deep breathing, music therapy, distraction) is also sometimes helpful, particularly when used in combination with other strategies.

If your parent has chronic pain

- Look into the availability of relaxation programs – or find a tape or CD that directs an individual to learn these techniques.

- Express your empathy; telling your parent that you understand that it is difficult to live with chronic pain can be helpful.

- Check with the doctor about a referral to a pain clinic. These specialty clinics can help people learn techniques to deal with chronic pain.

- Note that many seniors do not report chronic pain, believing that nothing can be done. Do not let them "grin and bear it." Treatment can improve quality of daily life.

Useful Resource

National Advisory Council on Aging (NACA). *Stop the pain.* http://www.naca-ccnta.ca/expression/15-3/exp15-3_toc_e.htm

Back Pain

Back pain can result from a number of interrelated problems of the spine, nerve roots, muscles, or ligaments in the back. The most common are injuries and age-related degenerative changes in the disks and facet joints of the spine.

Low back pain affects both men and women and usually starts between ages of 30 and 50 due to work-related injury. Risk factors include heavy lifting, twisting, body vibration, and obesity.

Treatment

Treatment of back pain usually involves medication and education on ways to protect the back. Muscle relaxants may be used for a short time. Conditioning exercises are often recommended for persistent problems. Surgery to remove damaged discs is also sometimes performed.

If your parent has back pain

- Consider physical therapy. Check with your parent's doctor.

- Encourage gentle exercise such as Tai Chi.

- Help with the delivery of heavy items.

- Offer to help reorganize - keeping heavy items on lower shelves may be helpful.

- Remember that mobility is important. There was a time when doctors recommended complete bed rest for problems such as back pain. It is now clear that full bed rest, in many cases, will lead to further deterioration. Some movement will help – but encourage your parent to learn and respect his or her limits.

Useful Resource

The Chronic Pain Association of Canada.
http://www.chronicpaincanada.com

How to Manage Chronic Illness and Disability

Many older adults have survived serious problems such a stroke, but are left with physical disability. Disability can also result from the progression of chronic disease such as arthritis or heart disease. Changes in physical ability can disrupt everyday life and impact relationships, roles, and the ability to fulfill responsibilities.

What can be done? Here is some encouraging news – most disabilities in older adults can be improved with active rehabilitation, an approach that focuses on strengths, minimizes limitations, and maintains independence.

Exercise is an essential ingredient in the health of older adults. The benefits of exercise also apply to older adults with disabilities. Exercise is needed to maintain circulation, muscle strength, and range of motion. Some seniors with disabilities may require assistance to enable them to exercise. The use of mobility aids, such as walkers, canes, and bathroom bars can also be highly useful in maintaining independence. Be certain that such devices are installed and maintained properly.

If your parent has a chronic illness and/or disability

- Physical therapy may be helpful.

- Occupational therapists always emphasize "able" versus "disable" – many physical activities can still be available to a senior with a disability.

- Seek support. Look for local community groups of the associations and societies mentioned in this chapter.

- Seek diagnosis and treatment from reliable sources. When possible, look for professionals with specialized education.

- Ask the following:

     1. What is wrong?

     2. What treatment is available?

     3. What are the benefits and risks of having the treatment and not having the treatment?

Take Action

  ➤ Recognize that aging, even with the limitations of chronic illness, need not prevent your parent from being useful, and from experiencing joy and meaning in life.

  ➤ It is never too late to start – healthy practices will improve well-being at any age.

  ➤ Take care of the things that can make a difference in preventing further problems. Your parents can benefit from regular vision testing, hearing testing, dental care, and physical exams. Further, good nutrition, good shoes, safety in the home, and medication management can all help delay the onset of problems.

> ➤ Knowledge is power! Help your older family member know more about his or her own health.

> ➤ Seek help and guidance from healthcare professionals and self-help organizations. They can provide information about services and networks that are available in your community.

> ➤ If in doubt, err on the side of safety and seek medical attention.

CHAPTER ELEVEN

CHALLENGES OF MENTAL ILLNESS

Mental health is equally important as physical health for overall well-being. In Chapter Two, you read about several factors that promote healthy aging and life satisfaction.

Studies have suggested that personality traits are relatively stable as people age, and that some personality traits can contribute to mental and emotional well-being. For example, someone who was an optimist at age 30 will probably still be an optimist at age 80. And optimism has been correlated to healthy aging.

Questions answered in this chapter:

What is mental health?
What are common mental health problems?
    Depression
    Anxiety
What do we need to know about addictions?
What is dementia?
What can I do to provide support and assistance to family members with mental health problems?

What is Mental Health?

Mental health generally refers to an individual's ability to interact with other people, and with their environment in ways that promotes a sense of well-being. Mental health is both influenced by and influences the individual's sense of personal control, achievement of goals, and perception of quality of life. Mental health requires adaptation and the ability to cope with the tasks of life and the usual stressful situations that arise.

How can older adults maintain good mental health? Chapter Two discussed some of the factors that influence health, meaning both physical and mental health. Some of these, such as contact with family and friends and keeping a positive attitude are important to mental health. Briefly, good mental health is influenced in later life by many factors:

- personal history of mental health throughout life,

- ability to control one's emotions,

- resiliency to cope and adapt to life's stressors and the changing demands that occur as we age,

- personality characteristics,

- socio-economic factors such as financial security,

- and support from family and friends.

How Seniors Maintain Mental Health

In many studies, the majority of seniors describe themselves as happy. They are able to maintain their satisfaction in life, even in the face of losses, changes in roles and increasing physical health problems. Many do this through adaptability, modifying their goals and aspirations, being flexible in problem solving and altering their reactions to stress. Many older adults learn the skill of accepting the things that they cannot change. Others also choose to avoid situations that cause negative emotions. You have probably noticed at least one occasion when you and your siblings were very distressed about something involving your parents but they appeared to be calmly riding out the storm. While you were "calling them to action" they were advising "things will work out for the best."

If you are reading this book, it is likely that you appreciate the importance of family support for older persons, but are you also aware that contact with friends is essential for emotional health? Friendships may, in fact, be more important than family for morale and a sense of autonomy and self-reliance.

Loneliness

Loneliness and social isolation tend to increase as people age because their social networks decrease. Loneliness is thus more likely to affect the mental health of those over 85. Women are at risk because they live longer than men and are more likely to be widowed.

Loneliness is a subjective experience. A lonely person may or may not be alone; in fact he or she may appear to have many social contacts. The sense of loneliness is a personal feeling of dissatisfaction with the nature of relationships or the frequency of contact. Understanding the difference between loneliness and isolation becomes important, for example, when you talk to your parents about housing. Older people are encouraged to move into seniors' housing to avoid being lonely.

If you wonder whether your parent is feeling lonely, you could ask some of the following questions.

- Do you have a really close friend?
- Do you have someone to talk to about day-to-day problems?
- Do you enjoy the company of others?
- Do you have people that you can lean on?
- Do you have enough friends and acquaintances?

What are Common Mental Health Problems?

Some seniors enter later life with a history of serious mental health problems, including bipolar disorder, depression, problems with addiction, or schizophrenia.

An individual who has problems of mood or anxiety and depression early in life will probably have these concerns in old age. Others develop these mental health problems only in later life.

A mental health problem or disorder is defined as a medically diagnosed illness that impairs the individual's thinking, feeling, or relationships.   Like physical health problems, mental health disorders are common among the older population. It is estimated that 20% of those over 65 have a mental health disorder.

The most common disorders in later life are those of mood and anxiety.   Increasing age is associated with increasing incidence of dementia, particularly for those over 85.   As well, older individuals continue to experience persistent life-long disorders of psychosis, bipolar disorder, and schizophrenia.   Finally, alcohol and drug addiction occur either as a long-time problem, or emerge as a new problem.

Sadly, older persons with mental illness often do not receive treatment. Reasons that contribute to under-treatment include:

- ageism; assuming that the problems are due to age,

- the stigma of mental health problems; afraid to seek treatment and be labelled as "mentally ill,"

- making a diagnosis is more difficult because the symptoms may be different in the older person,

- the appearance of symptoms is complicated by physical health problems,

- and a lack of health professionals with specialized training in mental health and aging.

Depression

Depression is a mood disorder that affects women more than men. It increases the risk of death from physical illness and suicide, and contributes to cognitive decline in older adults.

Depression is caused by a number of biological and social factors. A thorough medical assessment is necessary to diagnose depression.

Although everyone can feel "blue" or "depressed" when experiencing unhappiness or distress, depression as an illness is more serious. It can last for months and interfere with daily living and relationships. Unfortunately, many people are reluctant to seek help because of the stigma and prevalent misunderstanding that overcoming depression is just a matter of will power.

Like many other seniors, your parent may not talk about feeling depressed. You can be alert to the signs and symptoms listed below. If you notice these warning signs, talk to your parent and encourage a visit to the doctor.

Signs and Symptoms of Depression
• Loss of energy, feeling tired
• Difficulty concentrating
• Difficulty making decisions
• Loss of interest in usually activities
• Changes in sleep and eating patterns
• Decreased sex drive
• Avoiding people or social situations
• Overwhelming feelings of sadness
• Feeling unreasonably guilty
• Thoughts of death or suicide

Depression may be an ongoing problem that has been present since earlier life or one that is new in old age. The experiences of multiple losses and adjustment to changing family roles, finances, and other changes in later life can contribute to depression. In addition, some prescription drugs can cause or worsen depression.

Treatment
Depression can be treated through psychotherapy and medication. Usually, antidepressant medication takes about a month to show effects, so it is important to support the older person during this period. Good nutrition and exercise can also improve mood.

Suicide
People tend to think of suicide as an issue for younger people; however, the risk of suicide is high in older adults, especially older men living alone. Other risk factors include bereavement, psychiatric illness, alcohol misuse, previous suicide attempt, physical illness, and unmanaged pain.

Seniors considering suicide many not give any signs. If you are concerned about any senior, contact a crisis or distress line for advice.

Anxiety

Anxiety in older adults is not well understood by the public and probably underestimated by health professionals. Anxiety is likely as common in seniors as in younger adults; however, it is less likely to be diagnosed and treated. The common symptoms, such as palpitations (heart flutters), and shortness of breath are difficult to distinguish from medical problems.

If you believe that your parent has anxiety, the best action that you can take is to encourage diagnosis and treatment.

Treatment

There are many strategies for combating anxiety. Medications and therapy can make anxiety far more manageable. Do not believe the old adage that "an old dog can't learn new tricks" – even for those seniors have had a life-long struggle with anxiety, treatment can greatly improve their quality of life.

If your parent has a mental health problem

- First, help to overcome the stigma of mental health disorders and encourage your parent to seek treatment.

- It is never too late to seek treatment – although a person's age may change the strategies and the drug treatments that are used.

- Because there are physical changes that accompany aging, try to have a geriatric psychologist or a geriatrician involved in the treatment.

- Recognize that depression and anxiety are illnesses – not character flaws.

- Do not look at a low mood as a normal part of your parent's aging. It is understandable that there may be some sadness with losses and declining health, but depression is not inevitable in later life.

Useful Resource

Canadian Mental Health Association. British Columbia Division. http://www.cmha.bc.ca/resources/visions/seniors

What do we Need to Know about Addictions?

Alcohol and drug dependency are significant health problems throughout the life span. As many as 250,000 seniors in Canada experience problems with alcohol use. Like other mental health problems, misuse and abuse of alcohol are often under-diagnosed. Both the individual and the family are likely to deny that a problem exists. Some family members might not raise the topic because of their own drinking habits. Others might feel hopeless because the problem is long standing and the senior has refused previous suggestions to seek help.

Long-term alcohol abuse increases the risk of multiple physical health problems. They include

- gastritis (inflammation of the stomach),
- cognitive impairment (dementia),
- falls and injuries (i.e. fractures),
- and depression.

If your parent has problems with addictions

Talking about alcohol or drug use problems is very hard to do. Many family members prefer to avoid the subject or to hope that the family doctor will address the issue. Perhaps it would be easier to start the conversation if the family had hope and optimism. Remember, these problems are common, so your family is not alone, and treatment can be effective. Many older adults are successful in overcoming these problems.

If you are going to talk about this sensitive topic, consider these suggestions from www.agingincanada.ca.

- Treat the person with dignity and respect.
- Be gentle and caring.
- Recall happy memories and the person's good qualities.
- Present the facts in a straightforward manner.
- And most of all, stay optimistic and hopeful. Many seniors are more successful in treatment than are younger adults!

Useful Resource

Alcohol, Medications and Older Adults.
http://pathwayscourses.samhsa.gov/aaac/aaac_1_pg3.cfm

What Is Dementia?

Alzheimer Disease and other Dementias

The term "dementia" refers to the progressive decline caused by brain dysfunction. This dysfunction is seen in many areas of brain function (or cognition) including poor memory, absent or impaired communication (speech, writing, understanding spoken words), inability to recognize sensory information (sights, sounds, words), and impaired decision-making and judgment.

There are many types of dementia, but Alzheimer disease is the most common type, comprising about 2/3 of all cases. "Cognitive impairment" is another term used to describe the syndrome.

People have become quite terrified of developing Alzheimer disease or dementia. In reality, healthy older adults experience only minor changes in cognitive abilities as they age. Someone who forgets keys or loses a pair of sunglasses is not exhibiting early signs of the illness. With advancing age, however, the chances increase that an individual might develop conditions that impact cognitive function. A large Canadian study conducted in 1994 found that 8% of all people over the age of 65 years met the criteria for dementia, and the prevalence increases significantly with advancing age. The incidence was

- 2.5% for those aged 65 –74 years

- 11% for those between 75 and 84 years

- 35% for those over 85

Many people with mild cognitive impairment can live at home and manage independently. As the disease progresses, however, the individual may require more personal care and support. Dementia is a key reason older adults move to an institution.

Early diagnosis is important. People with cognitive impairment want to participate in future planning as early as possible. There are new medications that can slow the progression of the disease if started in the early stages. *Cognitive Retention Therapy* ™ is a structured program of cognitive exercises designed for individuals in the early stages of dementia. See Useful Resources at the end of this chapter for more information.

Families can be proactive and plan ahead. They can talk about how they want to address some serious issues such as living arrangements. They can complete a personal directive, talk about handling financial affairs, and arrange for services and care when these are needed.

If your parent has dementia

- Learn everything you can about the form of dementia that has been diagnosed.

- Do not feel it's your job to "bring them back to reality."

- See if a day program is available – stimulation and cognitive activities can have a beneficial effect.

- See if a family member is willing to spend time with the senior to record family stories or make a video of the senior telling family stories.

- When a parent is suffering from dementia, you do not become their parent; you are a caregiver. This can be a very difficult and taxing role, so be aware of your energy and get help through respite care or a day program when it is available.

- If your parent requires long-term care in a facility, try to find one that is designed specifically for dementia care.

There is much more to know about dementia. If your parent is showing signs or has been diagnosed, contact the local Alzheimer Society.

If your family member moves into a long-term care centre, you might value the advice given by Peter Silin. (See Useful Resources.)

Warning Signs of Dementia

How can you distinguish between normal memory changes that occur with aging – and the more serious problem of dementia, such as Alzheimer's disease? If you are concerned, here are some things to watch for.

First, forgetting, including people's names and events, is common as we grow older. But forgetting that is accompanied by confusion may be a warning sign of more serious problems. And forgetting the names of family members or familiar places is not an expected change. Other warning signs include

Doing or saying things repeatedly.

Difficulty making simple everyday decisions or difficulty completing everyday tasks.

Appearing restless and agitated.

Withdrawing and doing nothing for extended periods of time.

Becoming stubborn and uncooperative (different from always being stubborn).

Talking to oneself in a way that does not make sense (in contrast to talking to oneself for company or as a long-standing habit).

If you are worried, seek medical help. There are underlying medical conditions that can cause these types of changes – and treatment can be effective.

Source: ElderWise Info Vol. 2: 1. Used with permission

Useful Resources

Alzheimer Society of Canada. http://www.alzheimer.ca

Cognitive Retention Therapy™ www.crt-intl.com

Peter Silin. *Nursing Homes: The Family's Journey.* Available through bookstores or www.diamondgeriatrics.com

Take Action

> Learn more about mental health and mental illness. Knowledge will help you to overcome any fears or negative beliefs that you or others in your family might have. The Canadian Mental Health Association is an excellent source of information. Visit the website http://www.cmha.ca or call the nearest office.

> If you think that your parent is suffering from depression or anxiety, encourage medical treatment. People at any age, even those over 90, can benefit from drugs or therapy.

> If your parent is experiencing drug or alcohol dependence, seek help. First, get more information for yourself and your family. Then, approach your parent, armed with information about assessment and treatment programs that bring hope to the conversation.

> If your parent has dementia, seek support for yourself and your family. If one parent is the caregiver and the other has dementia, support can be vital to maintaining the health of the caregiver. The local Alzheimer Society can provide information on services available in your community.

> Take care of yourself. Supporting a parent who has a mental health problem can be very challenging. Learn more about self-care in Chapter Five.

CHAPTER TWELVE

ACUTE HEALTH CONCERNS

Unlike chronic health problems, acute conditions occur suddenly, often without warning. Recognizing these acute problems is important in order to seek early treatment.

This chapter provides you with the general signs and symptoms of acute health problems. It also gives specific information on some of the more serious problems of heart attack, stroke, influenza, and pneumonia.

Falls present a major risk for older adults. Too often a fall causes a fracture and results in hospitalization. Prevention is vital for those seniors who want to continue to live in the community.

Questions answered in this chapter:

What are the signs and symptoms of acute health problems?
  Heart Attack
  Stroke
  Influenza
  Pneumonia
What can be done to prevent falls?
What are the risks of hospitalization?
How can I help my parent in hospital?

What are the Signs and Symptoms of Acute Health Problems?

Any sudden or abrupt physical change should be considered an indicator that something new is developing and warrants medical investigation.

In the older adult, the following require immediate action:

- acute abdominal pain or tenderness,
- a rapid decline in cognitive function and level of consciousness (delirium),
- unexplained changes in personality or behaviour,
- respiratory distress,
- possible heart attack (difficulty breathing, pale skin, weakness, chest pain),
- fainting or falling,
- and suicide attempt.

Note: Telephone Health Lines can provide useful guidance to support decision-making regarding signs and symptoms. Contact your local health authority or provincial government to find a health line in your area.

Heart Attack

As people age, they are at greater risk for developing coronary artery disease, also called ischemic heart disease. It occurs due to the narrowing of the arteries of the heart that provide oxygenated blood to the heart muscle. When the tissue does not get enough oxygen, it dies. This tissue death causes a heart attack or myocardial infarction.

Angina or chest pain is a classic warning sign; however, older adults, especially women, may not develop the typical symptoms. Instead, they may become restless, extremely tired, or confused.

Men over 45 years and women over 55 years and those with a family history of heart attack or sudden death before age 55 are at a greater risk of developing heart disease. Cigarette smoking, high blood pressure, and diabetes are the top three risk factors for heart attack.

Recognizing a heart attack
If you are with your parent and you think he or she is having a heart attack, call an ambulance. Early treatment is essential.

If your parent has had a heart attack
Following a heart attack, people are strongly urged to start a fitness program, quit smoking, and maintain a healthy weight. You can encourage your parent to follow these recommendations, but nagging does not work.

Useful Resource
The Heart and Stroke Foundation: ww2.heartandstroke.ca

Stroke

Stroke or "brain attack" is a sudden loss of blood flow to the brain. Ischemic stroke, the most common, is due to vessel collapse or blockage in the vessel. Hemorrhagic stroke is less common and is a rupture of blood vessels causing bleeding in the brain. Strokes can lead to permanent impairment in both cognition and motor function. Warning signs include light-headedness, dizziness, headache, and memory or behavioural changes. Facial droop, arm weakness and speech abnormalities are also signs. Symptoms depend on the area of the brain affected. Many stroke victims lose consciousness.

Risk Factors
Risk factors for stroke include some chronic health problems such as high blood pressure, diabetes, and arteriosclerosis. Smoking is an important lifestyle risk factor.

Recognizing a stroke

Knowing what causes a stroke is important, but knowing how to recognize it could save someone's life! Here is a simple test. (Cincinnati Prehospital Stroke Scale.)

The test involves asking the person three simple questions:

1. Ask the person to <u>raise both arms and keep them up.</u> A person having a stroke will be unable to lift both arms, or cannot keep both of them raised.

2. Ask the person to <u>smile.</u> A person having a stroke will usually have paralysis or numbness on one side of the face and be unable to produce a symmetrical smile.

3. Ask the person to <u>repeat a short sentence word for word.</u> A person having a stroke will have confusion or difficulty speaking.

If you believe that a person cannot perform any of these simple tasks, call an ambulance immediately.

Treatment

Ischemic strokes that are caused by a blood clot can be treated using a new medication that breaks up the clot. This treatment needs to happen within three hours of the stroke. Other medical treatments include the use of medications called "blood thinners."

If your parent has had a stroke

- If your parent suffers a major stroke, he or she will need rehabilitation to regain lost function. Your support and encouragement will play an important role in recovery.

- Even a minor stroke can affect a person's thinking. Having patience and empathy can show that you understand.

- Recovery from a stroke can take time. Keep hope alive.

Influenza

Influenza is a viral respiratory infection caused by numerous strains of viruses.

At first, flu might look like a cold with runny nose, sore throat, and dry cough. Unlike a cold, however, the onset is usually quick and severe with symptoms such as fever, chills, lack of appetite, extreme weakness, and generalized body pain.

The flu, or influenza can have dire consequences for the older adult. Pneumonia is one serious complication.

Treatment

The most effective treatment is rest and plenty of fluids. Antibiotics do not treat viral infections.

If your parent has influenza

Before infection

- Encourage your parent to avoid crowds during flu season. Influenza is contagious.

- Talk to your parent about annual flu shots. Each year, the World Health Organization identifies the three strains predicted to be most common. The vaccine is made from these strains and therefore must be given every year.

During Infection

- Encourage bed rest and lots of fluids.

- Ask the pharmacist or physician for recommendations for over-the-counter medications to treat headache, fever, and muscle aches.

- Encourage your parent to seek medical treatment if symptoms worsen, or do not subside after a few days.

Useful Resource

Canadian Coalition for Immunization Awareness and Promotion. (CCIAP)

http://www.immunize.cpha.ca/english/index-e.htm

Pneumonia

Pneumonia is an infection in the lungs that may be caused by bacteria or viruses. It is a serious condition in the elderly. Older individuals are susceptible because of poor chest expansion, lowered resistance to infection, and conditions that cause reduced mobility.

Signs and symptoms of pneumonia are more difficult to detect in older adults, and a fever may not be present. Slight cough, fatigue, and rapid breathing may be evident. Confusion, restlessness, and change in behaviour may occur as a result of oxygen deficiency.

Treatment

If bacteria cause the infection, antibiotics can be used. Other treatment includes chest physiotherapy, fluids, and rest. The older adult may need to be in hospital.

If your parent has pneumonia

Before infection

- Talk to your parent about immunization. Pneumococcal vaccine is recommended for people over the age of 65. Some people will require the vaccine every five years.

During infection

- Encourage medical treatment if symptoms persist or worsen.

- If your parent has repeated infections, encourage medical treatment. Don't wait for the infection to become severe.

- Watch for other infections such as sinusitis or ear infections.

After an infection

- Encourage your parent to return to normal activities only at a slow and steady pace. It may take some time to be able to resume a regular day.

Useful Resource

Visit the website of the Canadian Lung Association and read about pneumonia in "Diseases A-Z." You can find the article at www.lung.ca or use the link below.

http://www.lung.ca/diseases-maladies/a-z/pneumonia-pneumonie/index_e.php

What can be done to Prevent Falls?

Falls are a significant risk in older people and one of the main causes of hospitalization. When they fall, older people are likely to suffer an injury, often a fracture or sprain. Falls cause more than 90% of all hip fractures in seniors, and 20% die within a year of this event. Almost half of admissions to long-term care facilities are as a result of falls.

Many risk factors contribute to falls:

- history of previous falls,

- depth perception challenges and vision problems,

- side effects of some medications,

- postural hypotension (drop in blood pressure when rising from a chair),

- and gait or balance difficulties.

If your parent is at risk to fall

- Raise the subject and talk about ways to reduce the risks, such as balancing regular activity / exercise with rest, and using proper footwear.

- Assess the home environment and ask to remove potential problems that may contribute to falls (clutter, scatter rugs, crowded furnishings, etc.).

- Become familiar with assistive devices such as canes, walkers, and bathroom grab bars.

- Encourage your parent to participate in exercise programs at senior centres or assisted living facilities. These programs can improve balance and strength.

- If your parent needs support when walking, learn how to provide assistance safely. Visit a home care and medical supply store and ask for instructions about safe ambulation. You can also contact a home care agency for information.

Useful Resource
The Public Health Agency of Canada at http://www.phac-aspc.gc.ca/seniors-aines has a wealth of information on falls in the elderly. Visit the home page and search for "falls." You can also find links to local prevention programs.

What are the Risks of Hospitalization?

Seniors, especially those over 75 years of age, are more likely than younger people to be hospitalized,. They also stay longer in hospital, on average 17 days, compared with less than 10 days for those under the age of 65.

The main function of acute care hospitals is to diagnose and treat acute illness or injury. But most conditions of elderly people are chronic and progressive, and their admissions to hospital are for "acute episodes of a chronic condition." While hospitalization may be necessary, there are potential risks including delirium, falls, bedsores, dehydration, constipation, deconditioning, and loss of functional independence.

The hospital setting focuses on efficiency, cost control, diagnosis, and treatment of acute illness and injury. Hospital environments are not always amenable to the care of older adults, which requires a more individualized approach that emphasizes coordinated care over time. In addition, staff shortages and lack of education regarding geriatric concerns is all too common in this setting. Let's look at two serious risks: delirium and deconditioning.

Delirium

Delirium is a term used for acute confusion associated with rapid changes in brain function. The person may become disoriented to time or place, and may be unable to concentrate or to speak. There may be a rapid alteration between being lethargic and agitated.

This problem is of particular concern for older adults, and should be considered a medical emergency. At the time of admission, as many as 10-22% of elderly patients are delirious, and as many as 20% will develop this condition within a few days.

Delirium has many underlying causes including infection and some medications.

Treatment

Delirium is sometimes overlooked in the hospitalized senior because the symptoms are similar to those found in dementia. If you notice signs of confusion in your parent, report this to the doctor or the nurse and ask questions about the possibility of delirium. Treatment depends on identifying the underlying cause.

If your parent has delirium

- Try to be present as much as possible. The presence of family members during hospitalization of older adults is invaluable. A friendly familiar face can help your parent to recover.

- Advocate for your parent. An older person experiencing delirium may not be able to inform hospital staff that these symptoms and behaviours are not typical but indicate a new problem.

- If you are unable to be there, recruit friends or hire a caregiver to attend. It is particularly important to be there to prevent falling.

Deconditioning

Deconditioning is another problem that affects seniors who are hospitalized, and it is caused by lack of mobility. Inactivity and bed rest can cause loss of muscle mass and strength. Deconditioning can occur in as little as two days on bed rest.

The human body is subject to the forces of gravity. Anyone who has watched a toddler learn to stand and walk can see the amount of strength it takes to pull even a little body up and to move it. Overcoming the force of gravity requires strength and energy. When a person is bedridden, gravity is not having its usual effect on the body. Without the force of gravity, the muscles and bones weaken. When circulation in the legs slows down, there is increased risk for blood clots. Moving, even taking small steps or performing little stretches, can make a big difference to recovery. The human body, even during an illness, is designed to be in some motion.

If your parent is at risk for deconditioning

- One of the best ways to maintain muscle strength and tone is to do gentle exercises. Ask if there are physical or recreational therapists available to teach your parent how to do safe exercises while lying in bed.

- Keep in mind that you do not want to push too far or take the attitude of "no pain no gain" with these exercises. They are meant to be gentle. Remember that some activity is better than no activity.

- For those who are well enough, simple range-of-motion exercises can be done while lying in a hospital bed. Generally, with a range-of-motion program, start at the shoulders and work through all the joints of the body, gently moving the limb through its normal range of movement. Make circles with the arms. Straighten and bend the elbow. Rotate the wrists. Open the hand and then make a fist.

- Even having the person sit up in bed a few times can help the muscles, since it requires multiple muscle groups to move from a lying position to a seated position.

If your parent is in hospital

- Family members need to take a strong advocacy role to speak on behalf of their parents.

- If possible, ask for healthcare providers who have specialized in Geriatrics or Gerontology.

- Ask questions and keep notes. Start a notebook or binder to keep track of people and information.

- Ask for a diagnosis and for an explanation of possible treatments. Be sure to find out the possible benefits and risks of the treatments.

- Obtain names of key contacts: head nurse, team manager, social worker, discharge planner, and rehabilitation therapists. Keep a list of phone numbers.

- Be prepared for transfers from the Emergency Room to an inpatient unit, and possibly to another unit as your parent's condition changes.

- Be prepared to be present at the hospital or recruit family and friends to be there. Consider hiring caregivers to give support and attention, particularly with personal care such as bathing, dressing, transferring, and eating.

Take Action

➢ Learn the signs of heart attack and stroke. You could save a life.

➢ Talk to your parents about vaccination for flu and pneumonia. Both conditions can have serious complications for older adults.

➢ Falls are serious. Use your influence with your parents to reduce the risks. If you do not have much influence, then recruit the support of others that your parents listen to such as the doctor, a good friend, or another relative.

➢ If your parent goes to hospital, do everything that you can to provide immediate support. If you cannot be there, try to find a substitute including friends, other family members, or paid caregivers. The risks for older adults are serious. Delirium could lead to a fall. Deconditioning can result in loss of function and inability to return home.

From the Authors

In Chapter Five, we quoted C. Eliopoulos.

> A family is a strong chain of human experience that bonds its members in life's challenges and joys.

We know that many of our readers enjoy their extended families, and they work well together. For them, supporting an aging parent is accepted as one of life's passages. We are also aware that others are not so fortunate, and they face greater challenges in trying to find "shared" solutions. In writing this book, we tried to be mindful of both types of readers. We wanted to offer many suggestions so that each family could find something of value to their unique situation. It is our hope that this book will serve as a useful guide for you and your family.

> I believe that getting the right information at the right time is the difference between making a good choice and making the best choice.

Maureen Osis

> I believe that the changing demographics of an aging society provide a compelling reason to build knowledge about healthy aging for everyone. The complex issues and dilemmas related to health, housing, and relationships can best be resolved by the generations working together to arrive at shared solutions based on sound, up-to-date information.

Judy Worrell

Notes

The authors wish to acknowledge the following sources of information, used to develop the book.

We also acknowledge the sources that were identified as "Useful Resources" throughout the book.

NOTE. For your convenience, all of the websites that are found in "Useful Resources" have been compiled into a document that can be found on the ElderWise website, www.elderwise.ca. Visit the Library page and look for "Useful Resources found in 'Your Aging Parents."

Chapter One

R. Butler. Ageism: Another form of bigotry. *Gerontologist*. 1969, (9). 243.

G. Hochman. What's driving boomers·crazy: Therapists report on their most urgent problems today. *New Choices: Living Even Better After 50*. 1998, 38(2). 30-33.

K. Lasher & P. Faulkender. Measurement of aging anxiety: Development of the Anxiety about Aging Scale. *International Journal of Aging and Human Development*. 1993, 37(4), pp.247-259.

E. Palmore *Ageism: Positive and negative*. New York, NY: Springer. 1990.

E. Palmore *The Facts on Aging Quiz* (2 ed.). New York, NY: Springer. 1998.

Statistics on Canada's population taken from the following sources:

(a). Canadian Council on Social Development for the Division of Aging and Seniors. *Statistical snapshots*. 1999. Retrieved from

http://www.phac-aspc.gc.ca/seniors-aines/index_pages/publications_e.htm#stats

(b). N. Chappell E. Gee, L. McDonald, &M. Stones. *Aging in Contemporary Canada*. Englewood Cliffs, NJ: Prentice Hall. 2003.

(c). Statistics Canada. *Seniors at work: An update.* The Daily, Wednesday, February 25, 2004. Retrieved from www.statscan.ca

Chapter Two

G. Burdman. *Healthful Aging.* Englewood Cliffs, NJ: Prentice Hall. 1985.

NACA. Successful Aging. *Expression. Bulletin of the National Advisory Council on Aging.* 2004, 17(4).

American Federation for Aging Research. Retrieved from http://websites.afar.org/site/PageServer?pagename=IA_feat2

C. Rosenthal. "The comforter: Providing personal advice and emotional support to generations in the family." *Canadian Journal on Aging.* 1987, 6(3). 228-239.

Chapter Three

CNIB. *I can't see as well as I used to.* Retrieved from http://www.cnib.ca/eng/publications/pamphlets/see_well.htm

Public Health Agency of Canada Aging and Seniors. *Hearing Loss Info-sheet for Seniors.* Retrieved from http://www.hc-sc.gc.ca/seniors-aines/pubs/info_sheets/hearing_loss/index.htm

Public Health Agency of Canada Aging and Seniors. *Assistive Devices Info Sheet for Seniors.* Retrieved from http://www.hc-sc.gc.ca/seniors-aines/pubs/info_sheets/assistive/index.htm

VON. *Foot care: What you should know.* Retrieved from http://www.von.ca/english/english/education/footcare/footcare national pp.ppt

Public Health Agency of Canada Aging and Seniors. *How you can help parents use medications safely.* Retrieved from http://www.phac-aspc.gc.ca/seniors-aines/pubs/med_matters/intro_e.htm

Chapter Four

E. Arnold & K. Boggs. *Interpersonal relationships: Professional communication skills for nurses.* (4th ed.). Philadelphia, PA: Saunders. 2003.

C. Martin. "Bridging the generation gap(s)." *Nursing*, 2004, 34(12). 62-63.

S. Merriam. "Time as the integrative factor." In M. C. Clark & R. S. Caffarella (Eds.). An update on adult development theory: New ways of thinking about the life course). *New Directions for Adult and Continuing Education.* Winter, 1999, 84. San Francisco, CA: Jossey-Bass Publishers. 67-75.

K. Smola & C. Sutton. "Generational differences: Revisiting generational work values for the new millennium." *Journal of Organizational Behavior.* 2002, 23. 363-382.

Chapter Five

E. Arnold & K. Boggs. *Interpersonal relationships: Professional communication skills for nurses* (4th ed.). Philadelphia, PA: Saunders. 2003.

R. Bolton. *People skills: How to assert yourself, listen to others, and resolve conflicts.* New York, NY: Simon and Schuster, Inc. 1979.

C. Eliopoulos. *Gerontological Nursing.* Baltimore, MD: Lippincott, Williams & Wilkins. 2004.

B. McLeod. *And thou shalt honor: The caregiver's companion.* Santa Monica, CA: Wiland-Bell Productions. 2002.

Chapter Seven

V. Morris. *How to care for aging parents.* New York, NY: Workman Publishing. 2004.

Chapter Eight

J. O'Donnell, G. McWaters, & J. Page. *The Canadian Retirement Guide: A comprehensive handbook on aging, retirement, caregiving & Health.* Toronto, ON: Insomniac Press, 2004.

Chapter Nine

R. Hubele. Presentation at Seniors' Housing Forum, 2004.

Canadian Council on Social Development for the Division of Aging and Seniors. *Canada's Seniors: Statistical snapshots.* 1999. Retrieved from http://www.phac-aspc.gc.ca/seniors-aines/index_pages/publications_e.htm#stats

A. Mihailidis. *Seniors' Housing Update.* 2002. For more information on research conducted by Dr. Alex Mihailidis, visit http://www.torontorehab.com/research/mihailidis.htm

Chapter Ten

Statistics Canada for the Division of Aging and Seniors. *Canada's Seniors: Statistical snapshots.* 1999. Retrieved from http://www.phac-aspc.gc.ca/seniors-aines/index_pages/publications_e.htm#stats

Content on the common chronic health problems taken from

(a). C. Porth. *Pathophysiology: Concepts of altered health states.* (7th ed.). Baltimore, MD: Lippincott Williams & Wilkins. 2005.

(b). E. Briggs. "The nursing management of pain in older people." *Nursing Standard,* 2003, 17(18). 47-53.

Chapter Eleven

M. Beishuizen. *Topics in geriatrics: delirium, dementia, and depression.* A presentation for the Edmonton AGNA Chapter Study Group. February, 2006.

N. Chappell, E. Gee, L. McDonald, & M. Stones. *Aging in contemporary Canada.* Upper Saddle River, NJ: Prentice Hall. 2003.

C. Eliopoulos. *Gerontological nursing* (5th ed.). Philadelphia, PA: Lippincott. 2001.

P. Mason & R. Kreger. *Stop Walking on Eggshells. Taking Your Life Back When Someone You Care About Has Borderline Personality Disorder.* Oakland, CA: New Harbinger Publications. 1998.

C. Porth. *Pathophysiology: Concepts of altered health states* (7th ed.). Baltimore, MD: Lippincott, Williams & Wilkins. 2005.

Chapter Twelve

N. Chappell, E. Gee, L. McDonald, & M. Stones. *Aging in contemporary Canada.* Upper Saddle River, NJ: Prentice Hall. 2003.

C. Eliopoulos. *Gerontological nursing* (5th ed.). Philadelphia, PA: Lippincott. 2001.

A. Gillis & MacDonald. "Prevention: Deconditioning in the hospitalized elderly." *Canadian Nurse*. 2005, 101(6). 16-22.

J. Miller & S. Elmore. "Call a stroke code!" *Nursing*. 2005, 35(2). 58-64.

A. Mitchell. *Older adult: Falls and fall injuries*. A presentation for the Edmonton AGNA Chapter Study Group. January, 2006.

C. Porth. *Pathophysiology: Concepts of altered health states* (7th ed.). Baltimore, MD: Lippincott Williams & Wilkins. 2005.

Statistics Canada for the Division of Aging and Seniors. *Canada's Seniors: Statistical snapshots*. 1999. Retrieved from http://www.phac-aspc.gc.ca/seniors-aines/index_pages/publications_e.htm#stats

Acknowledgements

The authors wish to thank our families and friends who supported us through this venture.

We also extend our appreciation to the many manuscript readers who shared their wisdom and advice.

Index

About the Authors
Maureen   Osis

is both a Registered Nurse, and a Registered Marriage and Family Therapist. As a gerontological professional she devoted her career to working with seniors and their families.

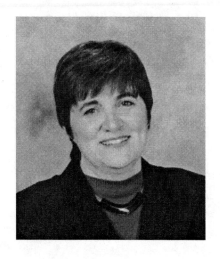

Maureen is a guest on television and radio programs that discuss aging and family dynamics, including "A New Look at Aging" on the Learning Channel.

Maureen is the co-founder of ElderWise Inc., a company dedicated to helping busy adults, seniors, and professionals find information and support on practical matters – like healthcare and housing, as well as the more delicate challenge of relationships between the generations.

Judy Worrell is a Registered Nurse, and throughout her career she has had consulting and educational roles in organizations that provide care to older people. She has worked in acute care, community health, home care, continuing care, and nursing education where she has pursued excellence in gerontological nursing practice.

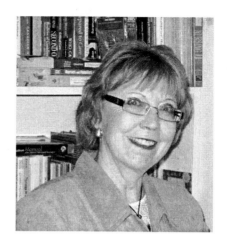

Judy is currently a Principal in Affinity Consulting, an Edmonton based consulting and training organization, and she is pursuing a Master of Nursing degree.

ISBN 142510796-6

9 781425 107963